THE EVOLUTION OF ETHICS IN AMERICA

In this book, Laurence Armand French frames the emergence of medical, clinical, and legal ethical standards within the long history of institutional and systemic racial and gender biases in the United States. He explores the role that White privilege and elitism play in justifying long-held discriminatory practices ranging from the eugenics crusade a century ago to the #MeToo and Black Lives Matter (BLM) movements of today. This book identifies and analyzes events highlighting systemic racism in the United States and explores how these events were exacerbated during the presidency of Donald J. Trump.

The evolution of ethical standards in the United States is a reaction to long-held practices that discriminate against certain classes of people based on gender, age, and race and ethnicity. The White supremacist worldview contributed to systemic biases that directly affect people of color as well as women, and those biases, in turn, are inherent components of the social structure of economic, academic, and judicial institutions. This process impacts both procedural and social justice, the very foundation of ethical standards of which our Constitution is based. This work attempts to unravel the social and psychological aspects of human behavior contributing to this phenomenon.

This concise yet comprehensive book is a valuable resource to a broad audience, including students of criminal justice, as well as scholars, researchers, and professionals in both the social and physical sciences.

Laurence Armand French has a Ph.D. in sociology (criminology)/social psychology from the University of New Hampshire-Durham; a postdoctorate in minorities and criminal justice education from SUNY-Albany; and a Ph.D. in educational psychology and measurement/cultural psychology from the University of Nebraska-Lincoln. He is Professor Emeritus of Psychology from Western New Mexico University and is currently an affiliate professor of justice studies, college of liberal arts, University of New Hampshire. He has also taught at HBCU facilities (Prairie View A&M University; Grambling University) and is widely published in the areas of minorities and social justice.

THE EVOLUTION OF ETHICS IN AMERICA

Standards Born of Crises

Laurence Armand French

Routledge
Taylor & Francis Group
NEW YORK AND LONDON

First published 2022
by Routledge
605 Third Avenue, New York, NY 10158

and by Routledge
2 Park Square, Milton Park, Abingdon, Oxon OX14 4RN

Routledge is an imprint of the Taylor & Francis Group, an informa business

Library of Congress Cataloging-in-Publication Data
Names: French, Laurence, 1941– author.
Title: The evolution of ethics in America : standards born of crises /
Laurence Armand French.
Description: New York , NY : Routledge, 2021. |
Includes bibliographical references and index.
Identifiers: LCCN 2021025076 (print) | LCCN 2021025077 (ebook) |
ISBN 9781032124148 (hardback) | ISBN 9781032123332 (paperback) |
ISBN 9781003224426 (ebook)
Subjects: LCSH: Ethics–United States–History.
Classification: LCC BJ352 .F74 2021 (print) |
LCC BJ352 (ebook) | DDC 170.973–dc23
LC record available at https://lccn.loc.gov/2021025076
LC ebook record available at https://lccn.loc.gov/2021025077

ISBN: 978-1-032-12414-8 (hbk)
ISBN: 978-1-032-12333-2 (pbk)
ISBN: 978-1-003-22442-6 (ebk)

DOI: 10.4324/9781003224426

Typeset in Bembo
by Newgen Publishing UK

CONTENTS

ACKNOWLEDGMENTS

This work reflects an unanticipated outcome of my Fulbright Specialist assignment at the Universidad Autonoma Indigenous de Sinaloa (UAIS) in Los Mochis in the fall of 2019. Two prominent community members, Mario Alvarez, M.D., Anaesthesiologist, and Ernesto Guerra Garcia, Ph.D., Coordinator of Graduated Studies at UAIS, were instrumental in involving me in their ongoing "ethics" group that eventually led to my presentation, "Evolucion de la Bioethica en Estados Unidos" at the Facultad de Enfermeria at the Universidad Autonoma de Sinaloa in Los Mochis on October 10, 2019.

My colleague Magdaleno Manzanrez at Western New Mexico also shares credit for this effort in that it was his collaborative efforts with Mexican institutions of higher education that led to the Fulbright assignment in the first place. He was instrumental in getting Dr. Ernesto Guerra Garcia at UAIS and Dr. Eva America Mayagoitia Padilla at the National Pedagogical University of Chihuahua to provide chapters for the 2019 *Routledge Handbook on Native American Justice Issues.* The handbook subsequently led to the Fulbright Specialist assignment at the Indigenous University in Los Mochis.

1

INTRODUCTION

> *Ethics* (a) The discipline dealing with what is good and bad and with moral duty and obligations; (b) A theory or system of moral values; (c) The principles of conduct governing an individual or group.[1]
>
> *Deontology:* The theory or study of moral obligations.[2]

Ethical issues are currently of both national (United States) and international concern ranging from crimes against humanity, human subject experiments, to sex abuse and human trafficking. Paramount to these concerns are institutional cover-ups and justifications for these actions by institutions of trust such as religious/sectarian groups, law enforcement agencies, educational institutions, and even the Boys Scouts of America. Historically shrouded in philosophical polemics, within esoteric academic or theological settings, deontological ethnics is often presented as a manifestation of man's (humans) *free will* or as an element of superior intellectual reasoning allowing for the pretense of superior paternalism by those who prescribe these ethical and moral standards for others. Often those providing these ethical and moral insights cite a higher authority with whom they have a privileged affiliation or refer to their self-proclaimed superior intellect as the source of their proscribed rules and logic supportive of their moral imperatives. Prophets and philosophers conjure up the "rights" and "wrongs" for human groups sharing a common ideological and cultural ethnomethodology. Examples are the "Ten Commandments"—the moral foundation of Judaism, Christianity, and Muslims. Another example is the "Hippocratic Oath" of "Do No Harm," the foundation of medical and clinical professions.

While seemingly universal in their application, cultural/worldviews differences come into play relevant to the distribution of these standards. Social psychological group dynamics such as "social stratification," "audience effect," "in-group/out-group dynamics," and the "confirmation/attribution biases" are crucial to any viable study of societal norms and values. While certain moral standards appear to be universal, such as the "Ten Commandments" or variations of this theme, their application is not absolute across cultural divides, or time, given that societal values are based upon the acceptable rules and their distribution at any given time. In this sense, societies are seen as artificial constructs subject to change over time. Accordingly, the acceptable rules, norms, and values are subject to change that need to reflect the group's prescribed epistemology at any given

DOI: 10.4324/9781003224426-1

time. All societies, past and present, have some form of stratification or hierarchical system of privilege even those that proclaim to be equalitarian in design. This is the case regarding sectarian doctrines that dictated social status according to a religious doctrine such as the Roman Catholic precept of *Original Sin* or the Protestant concept of *Divine Predestination*.

Given that societies are rarely static for long, the rules regarding acceptable behavior are also in flux. Here, the concept of "boundary maintenance" comes into play. Customs and laws dictate the acceptable norms at any given time maintaining a social and psychological boundary to guide members of the group and their position within the social structure. Rules often vary according to one's place within the social strata. The ones at the top usually are afforded privileges not shared by all members of the group often creating relative deprivation among the "have nots" or *the others*—out-group members. These rule makers, those establishing the group's acceptable boundaries, are generally at the top of the social strata hierarchy and are usually male, hence the "gender" factor. Accordingly, they often make rules that ensure their privileged position with the social structure. Race and ethnicity also play a significant role in the scheme of social class and privilege with *White supremacy* dominating the Euro-American social structures. The preamble to the U.S. Constitution is a prime example:

> We the People of the United States, in Order to form a more perfect Union, establish Justice, insure domestic Tranquility, provide for the common defense, promote the general Welfare, and secure the Blessings of Liberty to ourselves and our Posterity, do ordain and establish this Constitution for the United States of America.[3]

This proclamation has evolved greatly since first introduced in 1787 through amendments to be more inclusively relevant to gender, race, and class. Originally, it was meant only for White privileged adult males, many who owed Black slaves.

A measure of social justice is the application of rules, and their enforcement is to differentiate between the rules (procedural justice) and their application (distributive Justice) relevant to the society in general. This formula is also used to measure ethical standards and their enforcement. Rules are often codified into laws along with corresponding penalties, including consequences for violating professional ethics. Yet, the enforcement of laws and rules often varies greatly depending upon one's position within the social strata (privileged elite vs. social outcasts). Much of this difference between judicial ideas and the rule of law lies in the labeling of members of society as "insiders" (in-group) or "outsiders" (out-group). Georg Simmel, the German sociologist, put forth a theory of group dynamics that captures the friction between competing groups as they adjust to challenges to the status quo.

Basically, Simmel stated that changes to the status quo, the social boundaries which we are accustomed to, often lead to reciprocal antagonisms whereby hostilities and/or animosities directed toward a defined "out-group" serve to increase "in-group" cohesion. This formula works at both the domestic and international levels creating chaos, including wars, to distract the populace from economic or social unrest at home and to distract attention from internal problems.[4] Israel and Palestine both benefit from their seemingly perpetual reciprocal conflict drawing attention from serious domestic issues. Even then, the ethics of war has evolved considerably since the establishment in 1907 of international rules governing wars known as The Hague Convention. These rules address the brutal treatment of the Boer (Dutch) by the British in South Africa during the Boer War as well as the atrocities attributed to U.S. military forces in the Philippines in the aftermath of the Spanish American War. Both World Wars of the 20th century added to the "war ethnics" prohibitions as did the atrocities, including "brain washing" during the UN Korea Police Action (e.g., Korean War) and the blanket bombing and use of chemical defoliants and Napalm and other chemical weapons during the Vietnam War, leading to new prohibitions against chemical weapons and crimes against humanity, including genocide. The abuse of prisoners of war or civilian captives led to the Nuremberg Code of 1947 prescribing an "International Code of Ethics." Indeed, the Ten Points of the Nuremberg Code provide the basis of bioethics.[5]

1. The voluntary consent of the human subject is absolutely essential.
2. The experiment should be such as to yield fruitful results for the good of society, unprocurable by other methods or means of study, and not random and unnecessary in nature.
3. The experiment should be so designed and based on the results of animal experimentation and a knowledge of the natural history of the disease or other problems under study that the anticipated results will justify the performance of the experiment.
4. The experiment should be so conducted as to avoid all unnecessary physical and mental sufferings and injury.
5. No experiment should be conducted where there is an *a priori* reason to believe that death or disabling injury will occur; except, perhaps, in those experiments where the experimental physicians also serve as subjects.
6. The degree of risk to be taken should never exceed that determined by the humanitarian importance of the problem to be solved by the experiment.
7. Proper preparations should be made and adequate facilities provided to protect the experimental subject against even remote possibilities of injury, disability, or death.
8. The experiment should be conducted only by scientifically qualified persons. The highest degree of skill and care should be required through all stages of the experiment of those who conduct or engage in the experiment.
9. During the course of the experiment the human subject should be at liberty to bring the experiment to an end if he (she) has reached the physical or mental state where continuation of the experiment seems to him (her) to be impossible.
10. During the course of the experiment the scientist in charge must be prepared to terminate the experiment at any stage, if he has probable cause to believe, in the exercise of the good faith, superior skill and careful judgment required of him (her) that a continuation of the experiment is likely to result in injury, disability, or death to the experimental subject.[6]

Currently, a major focus on professional ethics is that of bioethics—the ethics of biology and medicine. Fritz Jahr, a Protestant German theologian and academician, is credited with coining the term in 1926, which coincidentally coincided with the eugenics movement in America and Europe.[7] Bioethics also overlapped with sectarian morality especially when addressing issues such as abortion, assisted suicide, circumcision, euthanasia, gene therapy, human genetic engineering, infertility treatment, life support, lobotomies, medical torture, organ transplants, pain management, pharmacogenetics, population control, psychcosurgery, reprogenetics, sex reassignment therapy, sperm/egg donation, stem cell research, sterilization, suicide, and transsexuality. Obviously, *professional ethics* is a major component of bioethics. And while bioethics is often dictated by law, professional ethics often adheres to a higher standard of practice within a specific professional occupational disciplines. A major challenge is when there is conflict between the law and one's professional ethics such as a journalist jailed for not disclosing a confidential source. A similar challenge is when an institution or discipline closes ranks in order to cover up individual or systemic ethical abuses. The *code of silence* phenomenon has been prevalent in recent cases, notably involving law enforcement agencies and academic institutions. Moreover, "whistle blowers" are often punished or otherwise ostracized for their actions given that it tends to brings bad press to the organization regardless of its proclaimed ethical standards. Given the institutional shroud of silence and opposition to external reviews, legal actions are often the only remedy to correcting these abuses, hence drawing even greater attention to institutional and/or individual abuses that otherwise could have been minimized through transparency.

The Human Dynamics of Law, Ethics, and Morality

Given that there are no universal moral imperatives, even regarding homicide, societies base their rules of conduct on the acceptable shared metaphysics explaining the "categories of understanding"—life and death, time and space, essence and being. This shared delusion, in turn, establishes the groups' "world view"—the perspective from which they judge themselves and others, in essence the foundations of their *ethnocentrism*. While many noted philosophers and theologians have presented complex argument regarding the moral foundations of societies, sociologist Erich Goode made as compelling and concise an argument as anyone, in my estimation:

> All civilizations set rules concerning what is real and what is not, what is true and what is false. All societies select out of the data before them a world, one world, the world taken for granted, and declared that to be the real world. Each one of these artificially constructed worlds is to some degree idiosyncratic, unique in itself. No individual views reality directly, in the raw, so to speak. Our perceptions are narrowly channeled through concepts and interpretations. What is commonly thought of as reality, that which exists, or simple is, is a set of suppositions, rationalizations, justifications, defenses, all generally collectively agreed upon, which guides and channels each individual's perception of the universe which man inhabits are more or less arbitrary, a matter of convention. Every society establishes a kind of epistemological methodology.[8]

Given the relative nature of our existence, we need to know our position within the social structure at any given time; who we are in relation to others within the group from which we glean our identity, our *persona*. It is within the hierarchy of the existing social stratification that we are assigned our relative status and corresponding roles, privileges, and entitlements within the group. All members of the group have to be cognizant of the social structure for these labels to have any significance. This is the case even in the most divided and structured hierarchies. Caste and class has significance only if everyone buys into the status quo. Even those on the lowest rungs of the social ladder must inculcate the status structure for the society to function; this is known as the "audience effect."

Social stratification is clearly articulated within the in-group, those we most want to impress—our reference group—while a more generalized stigmatizing status is assigned to out-groups. Out-group stigma often involves a blanket negative label that demonizes them and is a rallying call for in-group cohesion. It is within this context that the attribution or confirmation bias operates. This is a basic human phenomenon whereby the brain needs to simplify choices into a binary process much like the basis for artificial intelligence. Humans seek to avoid cognitive dissonance especially during times of crisis. In these situations, the more deliberative process of rational discrimination is replaced by a more visceral process of "gut" judgments based upon often highly charged sentiments and out-group labels. The mechanisms of the attribution bias are that we tend to rationalize or excuse bad behaviors of members of our group while overemphasizing these attributes among members of the out-group. This behavioral phenomenon operates at both the individual and group (collective) levels. The collective attribution biases reflect the group's rationalization and superiority (ethnocentrism) vis-à-vis that of the out-group. Hence, if someone within our group (in-group) succeeds at a task, we tend to attribute the success to inherent qualities, while, on the other hand, if someone on the out-group succeeds along similar lines, we tend to attribute this to external factors such as luck or unfair advantages. Accordingly, if someone in the out-group fails, or is caught doing something bad or illegal, we tend to attribute this to inherent factors, while attributing external excuses for a similar action afflicting in-group members.

Social norms and rituals further articulate the acceptable roles for its members regardless if they are labeled as being "insiders" or "outsiders." With this comes the process of legislating morality, whereby the power brokers within the society make rules that tend to maintain their control over others—maintaining a "self-fulling prophecy." This process is needed to maintain the social boundaries from which they continue to sustain their privileged position within the society. Accordingly, this process also occurs within the political realm (legislating morality) especially where different factions vie for control of the social agenda.

Contravening Ideological Perspectives and Moral Judgment

Taking Goode's thesis of shared constructed realities being the basis for social norms at any given time, Sigmund Freud addressed the role of religion within this scheme of things.

In his 1927 thesis, *The Future of an Illusion,* Freud postulates that religion is a shared illusion used to justify the collective social structure comprising a society:

> (T)he benevolent rule of a divine providence allays our fears of the dangers of life; the establishment of a moral world-order ensures the fulfillment of the demands of justice, which have so often remained unfulfilled in human civilization; and the prolongation of earthly existence in a future life provided the local and temporal framework in which these wish-fulfillments shall take place. Answers to the riddles that tempt the curiosity of man, such as how the universe began or what the relation is between body and mind, are developed in conformity with the underlying assumptions of this system.[9]

Contravening ideologies, sectarian or secular, are futile grounds for extreme actions directed against the group's perceived enemies. Simmel noted that intense intergroup antagonism follows two paths—calculating or spontaneous. Either way, the intensity associated with ideological and epistemological radicalism primes the groups for conflict and aggression; each group justifying their actions according to their group's ideals. Simmel termed calculating antagonism as *realistic conflict* reflecting action directed toward tangible social objectives such as status, power, and coveted resources. Spontaneous conflict, on the other hand, stems primarily from social frustrations that served to exacerbate the social divide within or between groups. This is called *non-realistic conflict*.[10]

According to social theorists, interpersonal, intragroup, and intergroup conflicts are inherent features of human coexistence given society's constant potential for change. Moreover, the dominant group within a society often sets the rules that benefit their continued authority over others within the social structure, including determinants of class, gender, religion, race, and ethnic standings. Rules and social control mechanisms are designed to favor maintaining the *status quo* and the privileged elite establishing the format for one's place in society, *knowing one's place.* Ostensibly, rules, such as laws, are made mainly for those highest on the social ladder, while a double standard exists for the lower classes. Rules for the prestigious in-group often call for humane treatment of its members while these standards are often diluted for the "lesser" groups. People at the extreme end of the social continuum are often labeled as non-humans therefore subject to inhumane treatment. Intergroup divisions are often predicated upon ideological differences both within the society and between competing societies: capitalism versus communism, Catholic versus Protestant versus Judaism versus Islam along with further subdivisions such as Roman Catholic versus Orthodox Christians and Protestant, Jewish, and Islamic divisions, each vying for a superior position within their respective societies. The inherent tensions within these intragroups manifest themselves in a number of ways including, at their most extreme, wars. The latter is reflective of Simmel's tenet of reciprocal antagonisms. This phenomenon can involve severe human atrocities whereby each group demonizes the *other,* relegating to inhuman status worthy of enslavement, ethnic cleansing, torture, massacres, and even cultural and physical genocide.[11]

Within this perspective, it is generally recognized that the Euro-American ideology, especially that which rationalized and justified the colonial era, especially the period from the late 15th century to the mid-20th century, was clearly based on *White Male Supremacy.* The corresponding ideology was rooted mainly in two contravening sectarian belief systems: Roman Catholicism and Calvinistic Protestantism. An overly simplistic interpretation of Catholicism is that it assigned a single status to its congregation predicated upon the belief that people were born with *original sin* and *free will* and that life itself was a trial of choosing between good and evil, the process relevant to obtaining absolution from the inherent stigma of original sin. Failure to earn or receive absolution of the original sin resulted in going to "Hell" or spending some of the "ever after" in "Purgatory." The ultimate reward being entry into "Heaven." Being predisposed with original sin life was a trial of good versus bad challenges with a preponderance of one over the other, along with adherence to the proscribed sacraments determining one's place in the hereafter. Thus, Catholicism is akin to communism, albeit a sectarian form of political Communism, whereby everyone's soul is perceived as being equal under God with one's behavior regulated by an elite supervisory hierarchy with special status and authority.

With the Protestant Reformation, notably *Calvinism*, a new worldview emerged based on the tenet of *moral predestine superiority*, a process that would become evident by one's earthly successes. Within this new *Protestant Ethic*, a predestined male would be identifiable to others in society by certain virtues: elevated social status, private wealth, and asceticism. Max Weber, the noted 20th-century scholar, articulated the link between Protestantism and capitalism. Here, Weber associates the emergence of capitalism with the Protestant concept of *predestination*, a marked contrast with the Catholic concept of *original sin*. This change in the Christian worldview was associated with the introduction of new Protestant religions—Calvinism, Pietism, Methodist, and the Baptist sects.[12]

On the surface, it could be argued that there were few differences between the sectarian doctrines of the Church of England (Anglicans) and those of the Roman Catholic Church other than the Head of the Church; this was not the case in the New World colonies. French, Portuguese, and Spanish colonies remained Roman Catholic, while the English colonies were Protestant. The Catholic perspective on the New World populace stemmed from Pope Julius II's decree of 1512 declaring that American Indians descended from Adam and Eve just like their White counterparts. England held a similar view treating Indian tribes as sovereign nations based on Anglican and Episcopal doctrines. The major departure came from the New England colonies and their more rigid and intolerant views regarding *others.*

While all the 13 British colonies engaged in the slave trade in one fashion or another, it was the Puritans that linked White elitism with the Protestant *Covenant of Divine Providence* as a justification for its rabid intolerance of other denominations and race and ethnic groups. This ideology differs markedly from the religious tolerance narrative spun around the Pilgrims. The emerging United States had its auspicious beginning as a business capitalist endeavor contracted with the British government. The Massachusetts Bay Colony was chartered as a business corporation with legal authority to exercise law and order among its inhabitants. These Crown Charters were managed by an appointed governor, deputy governor, and a board of stockholders, known as "freemen." The freemen constituted a "general court" tantamount to a legislature that met four times annually in order to conduct corporate business such as admit new members, elect officers, and make rules and regulations. Religious tolerance was not a part of the Massachusetts Bay Colony. Indeed, the Puritan leaders held an elitist view of Protestantism whereby only selected male members were enfranchised. Until 1630, church membership required a minister's endorsement, creating a strict social stratification even among free Whites. Women, indentured Whites and people of color (Blacks and Indians), suffered even more within this restrictive social milieu. Kai Erikson surmised the colonial Puritan's society as follows:

> God has chosen an elite to represent Him on earth and to join Him in Heaven. People who belonged to this elite learned of their appointment through the agency of a deep conversion experience, giving them a special responsibility and a special competence to control the destinies of others.[13]

The asceticism of the Puritans, in general, and their particular brand of Protestantism, the Congregationalists, in particular, fueled not only ethnocentric elitism but a ferocious hatred of anything they perceived as contrary to their beliefs. This included other Protestant sects, including the Church of England, and especially Catholicism and Indigenous belief systems. With blatant disregard for native occupants, the Congregationalists established their own theocratic communities (congregations), making each a separately constituted unit. Within this setting came the bloodletting against challenges to the New England Puritan theocracy, notably the Quaker persecutions of 1656–1665. Here, the anti-Quaker law carried the death sentence for anyone professing to be a Quaker within the Puritan colonies. Hence, the legislation of morality in America had its origins in the colonies. Divine Providence expressed itself in the concept of *Manifest Destiny*—the right over indigenous peoples to all the lands and resources in North America.[14]

The emergence of American jurisprudence has its foundation in Medieval Catholicism and its concept of *free will* in choices in life in order to absolve oneself from the stigma of *original sin*. Within this framework, serious infractions of the norms were deemed *mortal sins* and lesser offenses were termed *venial sins*. Culpability, or intent to do evil, was termed *mens rea*. The secular adaptation of this model resulted in mortal sins equating *felonies* and lesser sins being labeled *misdemeanors*. While American laws are said to be based upon British "common laws," this is mainly due to the fact that King Henry VIII basically retained the tenets of Catholicism with the exception of recognition of the Pope as head of the Church of England. America's statutory laws were based on this model with justice determined via a paternalistic adversarial trial process. American justice was a White male-dominated institution up until the latter half of the 20th century. Accordingly, equal justice, along with the caveat of *innocent until proved guilty beyond a reasonable doubt*, pertained mainly to adult White males. Women, children and adolescents, and racial and ethnic minorities were treated as classes of people that were subjugated to the "protection" and supervision of the ruling White male elite. The fallacy of this system was that the rules governing acceptable (legal) behaviors were often heavily slanted in favor of the ruling class hence creating a self-fulfilling prophecy that tended to perpetuate their "superiority" and the imposition of their moral imperatives such as women's rights, civil rights, and even the administration of the death penalty. Changes slowly came about through landmark court decisions based on civil rights protests as well as the advent of neuroscientific methods. This book explores the changing landscape of laws and ethnics as they have evolved within American society.

Notes

1 MA: Merriam-Webster Inc., p. 426.
2 *Ibid.*, p. 340.
3 See *The Constitution of the United States of America.*
4 Simmel, G. 1955. *Conflict* (Wolff, K.A., trans.). New York, NY: The Free Press.
5 See *Nuremberg Code of International Ethic*; Annas, G.J., & Grodin, M.A. (eds.). 1992. *The Nazi Doctors and the Nuremberg Code: Human Rights in Human Experimentation.* New York, NY: Oxford University Press.
6 *Ibid.*
7 See Sass. H.-M. 2007. Fritz Jahr's 1927 Concept of Bioethics. *Kennedy Institute of Ethics Journal*, Vol. 17 (4), pp. 279–295.
8 Goode, E. 1969. Marijuana and the Politics of Reality. *Journal of Health and Social Behavior*, Vol. 10, pp. 83–94.
9 Freud, S. 1927; 1964. *The Future of an Illusion* (Robson-Scott, W.D., trans.; Strachely, J., ed.). Garden City, NY: Doubleday Anchor.
10 See Simmel, op. cit. 4.
11 *Ibid.*
12 Weber, M. 1930. *The Protestant Ethic and the Spirit of Capitalism* (Parsons, T., trans.). London, England: Allen & Unwin.
13 Erikson, K.T. 1966. *Wayward Puritan: A Study in the Sociology of Deviance.* New York, NY: Wiley & Sons.
14 Stephanson, A. 1995. *Manifest Destiny.* New York, NY: Hill and Wang.

2

DUE PROCESS

The Ethics of Social Justice

Genesis of Institutionalized Racism in America

The American/Nazi Connection Regarding the Pseudo-Science of Eugenics

It is important to explore the historical antecedents leading to the abuses surrounding the notorious *Tuskegee Syphilis Study* and the corresponding forced sterilization of Blacks and American Indians within American society. Clearly, America's legacy of White supremacy was seriously challenged by the U.S. Civil War (War between the States) and the end of slavery, along with the onslaught of Asian laborers and non-Protestant emigrants, resulting in the need to reemphasize the moral superiority of the dominant White Anglo Saxon Protestant (WASP) society. The answer seemed to lie in the emerging scientific quest for human and social evolution, a movement based on *Social Darwinism* and eugenics.

The American Heritage Dictionary defines *eugenics* as the study of hereditary improvement of the human race by controlled selective breeding. The term itself stems back to the late 19th century with the British psychologist, Sir Francis Galton, cousin of Charles Darwin, who coined the term and proposed the science of eugenics in order to produce a highly gifted race. Galton's (1869) theory of social Darwinism and the creation of a superior race were widely supported in the United States during the early 20th century. Indeed, the concept of White supremacy in the United States dates back to its early history with the long-held concept of *manifest destiny*—that belief that White males were predestined by God to be superior to all others. The eugenics movement emerged during the late 19th and early in the 20th centuries both in Europe and the United States at the intersection of two movements—social evolution and mass immigration. This was especially the case in the United States which was challenged by the large influx of immigrants from southern and eastern Europe and Asia which led to the Dillingham Commission and the advent of immigration and border control in addition to restrictive quotas for those not from northern and western Europe. The thinking at the time was that a better quality of human beings could come about through social engineering, a movement endorsed in the United States by both politicians (namely Republicans, including Theodore Roosevelt, William Howard Taft, and Woodrow Wilson) and top scholars at the prestigious Ivy League colleges and universities. The general idea was that you could "breed out" undesirable human traits hence creating a better human race.[1]

DOI: 10.4324/9781003224426-2

The eugenics movement led to federal control over immigration and passage of a rash of immigration laws from 1882 until 1924 and beyond, including the infamous Chinese Exclusion Act of 1882 and the U.S. Supreme Court decision, *Plessy v. Ferguson*, that upheld racial segregation. An unintended consequence of the eugenics movement was that it emboldened racial and sectarian hate groups such as the Ku Klux Klan (KKK) with its florid racial and anti-Catholic and anti-Semitism rhetoric that accounted for decades of lynchings.[2] Nazi Germany later followed the United States in supporting the social engineering of a superior Aryan race. Clearly, eugenics and racism are closely associated providing a seemingly objective rationale for social discrimination along the lines of race, class, caste, and even gender. It fostered such practices as Apartheid, ethnic cleansing, and *genocide* (a concept coined in 1947 following the Nazi War Trials).

Blacks, American Indians, Asians, and other non-Whites and even non-Protestant Whites, as well as those determined to be mentally deficient were quickly labeled as being *genetically defective* and needed to be cleansed from the U.S. population. In Nazi-influenced Europe, the classes of human defectives included Jews, Gypsies (Roma), non-Whites, and even Whites not considered the genetic equivalent of northern and western European Caucasians such as Serbs. The Nazi atrocities were widely publicized due largely to the extremes taken in the *final solution*. What is less known is America's well-kept secret of sterilization, institutionalization, and execution of those deemed genetically inferior to the dominant White society. The White elite in U.S. society found a champion for their cause at Stanford University with psychologist Lewis M. Terman (1916) and his revision of the original 1908 French Binet–Simon IQ test.[3]

Lewis Terman was influenced by his mentor Francis Galton who was considered to be the founder of scientific psychology setting the stage for the use of psychological tests to implement the dictates of Social Darwinism. Eugenics, implemented partly through involuntary sterilization, was seen as the means for achieving successful Social Darwinism in the United States. The goal of eugenics was the improvement of the human race through the elimination of what were considered to be defective genes. It was Terman who provided the otherwise seemingly objective measure of determining who was unfit. Terman was confident that his version of the IQ test would accurately weed out the genetically deficient members of American society, what he termed the serious deviant. His solution included plans for eliminating these genetic inferiors through institutionalization and sterilization. Terman proposed his 1916 IQ test, the *Stanford-Binet*, as a scientific tool for determining those in society that needed to be controlled and eventually taken out of the gene pool. What was not factored into this test was the racial and class bias of his sample—the upper middle-class White faculty and families at Stanford University.

By 1926, 23 states had enacted compulsory sterilization laws and this practice was condoned by the U.S. Supreme Court in 1927 in its decision, *Buck v. Bell*.[4] This decision was based mainly on Terman's views:

> It is safe to predict that in the near future intelligence tests will bring tens of thousands of these high-grade defectives under the surveillance and protection of society. This will ultimately result in curtailing the reproduction of feeble-mindedness and in the elimination of an enormous amount of crime, pauperism, and industrial inefficiency … Not all criminals are feeble-minded, but all feeble-minded are at least potential criminals. That every feeble-minded woman is a potential prostitute would hardly be disputed by anyone … Considering the tremendous cost of vice and crime … it is evident that psychological testing has found here one of its richest applications.[5]

Of course, this assessment did not take into account the poor educational opportunities afforded to Blacks and other minorities in U.S. society under de jure and de facto segregation, mandated by laws and affirmed by the U.S. Supreme Court, hence further fueling existing discriminatory practices that not only produced substandard education but a biased measurement of someone's true intelligence. Also, the stigma associated with being genetically inferior led to harsh solutions for those falling into this category even if their only *societal offense* was procreation. It is estimated that over 60,000 individuals, mainly African American and American Indian females, were involuntarily sterilized in 35 states at both the state and federal levels (Indian Country is federally administered) until this practice was challenged during the Civil Rights era of the 1960s when it was disclosed that those most likely to be subjected to this practice were poor minorities. While California recorded the most cases (20,000), North Carolina continued this practice until 1974. While the practice of compulsory sterilization began to wane in the late 1960s and early 1970s, the practice of ethnic and genetic cleansing continued in U.S. society through other avenues most notably incarceration and the death penalty.

Barnes and Teeters noted that sterilization had its roots within the criminal justice system with the first operation being performed in 1899 at the Jeffersonville Indiana Reformatory.[6] The horrors of Nazi eugenics during World War II played a role in its demise in the United States. Nonetheless, the eugenics movement in the United States clearly contributed to the general stereotype of racial inferiority, a status often based on flawed testing, and the need to control these "inferior" human beings. In 1972, the controversy over the stigma associated with psychological testing came to a head in California, the state that led the country in forced sterilizations. The issue involved the use of standardized tests to label students within the California public schools as being mentally deficient, a stigma that followed them throughout their lives. It is interesting that Terman and his Stanford-Binet test played a significant role in this controversy. The legal case, *Larry P. v. Riles*, began in 1972 about the same time that forced sterilization was coming to an end and school integration was being forcefully implemented throughout the United States. Part of the problem with this unfounded stereotype was that it fostered the association between racial inferiority and mental deficiency, along with the potential for violence among this group. This stereotype continued to plague American society into the 21st century, leading to the *Black Lives Matter* outcry which was that these "inferior" people of color also had a greater potential for violence.[7]

The Emergence of America's Double Standard of Justice

Collective biases are imbued in human socialization and enculturation where we learn "our place," or standing, in society. We come to believe that brutality and hateful vengeance resulting in mass murder of unarmed civilians, rapes, torture (beheadings, genital mutilations, etc.), mass incarceration under dire conditions, and forceful expulsion from homes and communities, etc. are attributes associated with the lower tier, inferior peoples and not with the *civilized* superior elites. Yet, unfortunately, these are attributes common to civil wars regardless of race, class, or religion; a situation associated with collective fears and irrationalities. Indeed, the latter, sectarianism and political ideology, often serve to exacerbate the flames of intergroup fears and hatred leading to collective irrational behaviors, e.g., mobs, vigilantism, and riots.

Social norms, rituals, and laws further articulate the acceptable roles for its members regardless if they are labeled as being "insiders" or "outsiders." With this comes the process of legislating morality, whereby the power brokers within the society make rules that tend to maintain their control over others—maintaining a "self-fulling prophecy." This process is needed to maintain the social boundaries which they continue to sustain their privileged position within the society. Accordingly, this process also occurs within the political realm (legislating morality) especially where different factions vie for control of the social agenda.[8]

The Adversarial Justice Model

Justice, then, is a relative construct often influenced by geopolitics and ideology complicating any sense of judicial fairness or objectivity. Societies qualify what they term to be justice along with a prescribed method for administering justice. The contemporary Euro-American *Adversarial Judicial Model* is based primarily on the Christian (Catholic/Orthodox and Protestant sects) concept of "free will" where the individual is seen as being solely responsible for his/her actions. Here the crime is seen as a choice between "good" and "evil" whereby serious sins (crimes) are considered to be *mortal* (felonies) and lesser offenses to be venial sins (misdemeanors). The major issue being the individual's free choice to sin, hence the secular concept of *mens reas* (intent).

The secular process of determining one's intent is based on "game theory" whereby a prescribed set of rules are devised in order to determine how the game (trial) is to be conducted and what are the roles assigned to the players (prosecution, defense, judges). The justice game concept is based on the ideal that there is a level playing field and that the contestants are equally qualified to play the game. In this ideal scenario, the players (state/prosecution; defense/accused) have equal *standing* before the court while the judge and/or jury are expected to be neutral and value free. In essence, the justice game model is like other games with its focus not on "justice per se" but on "winning" the game. Scores are kept and careers enhanced or destroyed according to the judicial results. In certain instances, the results have life and death consequences. In reality, like sports, the judicial game often has a hidden agenda, that of appeasing the public audience. And whenever there is a hidden agenda, there is the tendency to deceive, in essence, to cheat thereby "tilting" the playing field.

Our focus is on the U.S. model given that America initiated and dominated the first major forum for international justice—the ad hoc war crime tribunals following World War II—the Nuremberg Trials and the International Military Tribunal for the Far East (IMTFE)—where the United States set the stage (articulating the rules of the game and deciding how level of the judicial field would be). The Americans ensured dominance over these judicial proceedings by providing the lead prosecutor in both tribunals. According to the U.S. model, the adversarial process involves a contest between two independent authorities, the prosecution and the defense, which ideally argue their case before a jury of peers in a scenario refereed by a neutral third party (judge) whose role is to make certain that the respective player follows the rules of the game. Appeals are based solely on contested rule violations and not on the juried outcome (innocence or guilt). Bench trials, on the other hand, occur when the defendant choses to forego the jury trial and take their chances with a sitting judge who supposedly determines innocence or guilt based on the evidence brought before the tribunal. Both U.S.-dominated World War II tribunals had judicial juries comprised only of members of the victorious nations in the conflict.

This process originates with the omission and reporting of a statutory violation, deemed criminal, followed by the following steps: indictment, arraignment, plea to charge, trial, verdict, sentence, and appeal if found guilty. Punishment, including severe retribution such as the death sentence, is then justified under this model. In the United States, the *due process* perspective is based on the presumption of innocence, thereby forcing the prosecution to present their case before a petit jury arguing the defendant's guilt *beyond a reasonable doubt*. Mechanisms have evolved in order to ensure that innocent parties are not summarily adjudicated guilty by fiat doled out by either government agents and/or sectarian leaders. *Habeas Corpus*, derived from British Common Laws, is designed to provide protection from unreasonable arrest, detainment, and severe punishment. Moreover, defendants are to be made aware of the charges against them, afforded defense attorneys, and made aware of their rights against self-incrimination as well as other guarantees such as warrantless search and seizures, excessive bail, and unreasonable detainment before trial. Defense attorneys are armed with the *discovery* process whereby they should have access to all the materials gathered by the prosecution prior to the advent of the judicial contest. Failure to provide these materials amounts to a major procedural error, one that warrants an appeal and the likelihood of a mistrial.

Amendments to the U.S. Constitution spell out these judicial ideals. The Fourth Amendment addresses *search and seizure,* guaranteeing the right of the citizens to be secure in their persons, houses, papers, and effects, against unreasonable searches and seizures that could be used against them in a court of law. This Amendment also stipulates that *probable cause* is a requisite for any warrant to search for and subsequently seize evidence that then can be introduced in court. Rights in criminal cases are guaranteed by the Fifth Amendment with protection against indictments of capital crimes without the benefit of a grand jury indictment. This Amendment also protects against double jeopardy and protects individuals from self-incrimination or being forced to be a witness against him/herself. Accordingly, individuals are not to be deprived of life, liberty, or property without due process of law; nor shall private property be taken for public use without just compensation. The Sixth Amendment of the *Bill of Rights* provides for the right to a speedy and public trial, by an impartial jury from the jurisdiction where the alleged crime was committed. Moreover, the accused needs to be informed of the nature and cause of the accusations and to have the opportunity to confront the witnesses against him/her as well as having access to adequate defense counsel. The Eighth Amendment calls for the protection from excessive bail and fines and protection against cruel and unusual punishment (U.S. Constitution).

Ideally, the U.S. criminal justice process originates with the commission and reporting of a statutory violation, deemed criminal, followed by arrest where the suspect is read the *Miranda warning* that they have the right to remain silent and to have a defense attorney present during any interrogation. Next comes the preliminary hearing in order to determine probable cause and intent (*mens rea*). Juveniles and adults with compromised mental capabilities are not thought to possess the capacity for mens rea. Once indicted, the charges are read in court at arraignment. Here, the defendant is asked to plea to the charges. A plea of *not guilty* signifies the exercise of one's right to a trail by a jury of their peers known as the petit jury. It is in this arena that the contest begins pitting the defendant against the State (prosecution) with a judge serving as referee and the final outcome determined by a jury of their peers. A guilty verdict is based on a unanimous decision by the jury (anything less leads to a mistrial) as against a preponderance of probability for civil cases. A guilty verdict is accompanied by the stigma of being a "convict" (felony or misdemeanor) and a criminal sentence seals that status. Sentencing is done by the presiding judge. While the verdict, per se, cannot be appealed, alleged procedural error can be as well as challenges to the proportionality of the judge's sentence to the offense for which the person was convicted.

Most criminal adjudications occur at the state level where the court structure includes the *inferior court system* where misdemeanors are processed before a bench while jury trials occur in the *superior court* system which generally are held at the county level and processed by the District Attorney's office. Defendants have the right to appeal inferior/bench trial misdemeanor decisions to the superior court and a jury trial. The next level of state courts is the appellate courts with the top court designated the State's *Supreme Court*. A similar hierarchy occurs at the federal level with the country divided into federal court districts. These courts are limited to federal laws which, for the most part, pertain only to Indian Country and federally controlled public lands. Here, the

U.S. Marshals, the Federal Bureau of Investigation (FBI), and a host of other federal law enforcement agencies have original police jurisdiction. Federal courts offer plea deals at the Magistrate Court level, while other federal cases are adjudicated before Federal District Trial Courts where juries are selected where the federal district is situated. Federal District Courts also serve as an appeal court for state cases once the state judicial system has been exhausted. Many of these cases address questions of Habeas Corpus appeals from prisoners. The next level of federal jurisdiction is the U.S. Circuit Courts of Appeals, while the ultimate court of the land is the U.S. Supreme Court.

Within this system, an individual charged and convicted for a state-level offense has the potential for appeal of his/her case to the highest federal court in the land. This is indeed an admirable system if practiced according to its ideals. While this model was originally designed only for enfranchised Protestant adult males (privileged elite) during the early years of the American Republic, it has been modified to be more inclusive now including all U.S. citizens regardless of age, gender, race, ethnicity, or religion. Adversarial and social justice are compatible when the laws (procedural justice) are applicable (distributive justice) to all those participating in the adjudication process. *Standing* before the court implies equal status among the participants—prosecutor representing the state; judge, juries (Grand and Petite), defendant, and defense attorneys.

Jim Crow Justice

Deviating from this formula often leads to a miscarriage of justice especially for those not enfranchised or other members of socially defined out-groups. Blacks (Freedmen) were not enfranchised until 1868 with the enactment of the 14th Amendment to the U.S. Constitution: "All persons born or naturalized in the United States, and subject to the jurisdiction thereof, are citizens of the United States and of the State wherein they reside … excluding Indians."[9] Black citizenship status changed dramatically 28 years later when the U.S. Supreme Court, in *Plessy v. Ferguson*, upheld the harsh Jim Crow segregation laws of the South officially sanctioning African Americans as "second-class citizens."

The infamous 1896 U.S. *Plessy v. Ferguson* case that adjudicated American Blacks as inferior to Whites, based on its decision against Homer A. Plessy, legally relegating them to permanent second-class citizenship and another 72 years of discrimination with license to intimidate, harass, and even kill indiscriminately. Ironically, judicial fiat often supersedes both legislative and executive authorities in that it provides the ultimate interpretation of these cases according to the prevailing constitutional and societal norms.[10] The *Plessy* case legitimized the so-called *separate-but-equal* (Jim Crow) status imposed on Blacks by the southern states that once comprised the Confederacy by upholding the constitutionality of racial segregation in the United States, a decision that empowered hate groups like the KKK and indiscriminate, unadjudicated lynchings (killing by hanging, burning, dismembering) of Blacks without the benefit of *Due Process*. It also justified the disproportionate imprisonment of American Blacks, an unfortunate legacy that continues to the present. Hence, this single decision overturned the fact that the Confederacy lost the Civil War; it allowed for the public display of Confederate monuments as constant reminders for both Blacks and Whites as to the supremacy of Whites over Blacks and other minorities of color—American Indians, Hispanics, Asians, increasing the open display of Confederate flags.

The proliferation of massive monuments soon prevailed following the *Plessy* decision with statues of Confederate military leaders dominating public and government buildings and parks as a constant reminder of the White's supremacy over those of color who were, in turn, subjected to inferior services, including education, within this social caste system creating a self-fulfilling prophecy that guaranteed their inferior status. These totems and monuments have only been challenged recently and taken down over a century since the *Plessy* decision. For all those years, statutes reflecting the leaders of the brutality of slavery, Jefferson Davis, Robert E. Lee, Stonewall Jackson, etc., were constant reminders of the inferiority of Blacks vis-à-via the superiority of Southern Whites. The *Plessy* decision emboldened the radical White right in America where today both the Confederate and Nazi flags are symbols of these hate groups. Indeed, the swastika, the most notorious symbol of hate worldwide, is used to identify neo-Nazi groups.

What is not commonly recognized in America's public/private educational curriculum is that "institutional racism" in the United States emerged as a clandestine agreement between Republicans and Southern Democrats following President Grant's administration. "Jim Crow" discrimination emerged during the disputed Hayes-Tilden presidential compromise of 1877 that essentially allowed Republicans to retain the White House in exchange for ending Reconstruction in the South. The mechanism for this was the transfer of federal civil protection (Due Process) for the newly freed Blacks to state authority, which was dominated by Whites, many who were Confederates or Confederate sympathizers. While the administration of Andrew Johnson bore the brunt of blame associated with Black disenfranchisement, the deal of Jim Crow discrimination was actually secured during the administration of President Rutherford B. Hayes (1877–1881) paving the foundation for the 1896 U.S. Supreme Court *Plessy v. Ferguson* decision.[11]

Jim Crow advocates were again charged up during the Woodrow Wilson administration (1913–1921) whose presidency did more to legitimize segregation, including banning Blacks from attending Princeton while the university's president. Interestingly, his racial views did not vary much from that of his White elite opponents in the 1912 presidential election, former president, Theodore Roosevelt (1904–1908) and William Howard Taft (1908–1912). The main difference was that Wilson formally instituted segregation at the federal level in concert with the Jim Crow South. Wilson stacked his administration with conservative southerners including Treasury, Agriculture, Attorney General, Secretary of the Navy, and Postmaster General—all willing agents of White supremacists. Wilson's racists sentiments gained national attention on February 18, 1915, when he held a private viewing for this cabinet members and their families of the inflammatory film, *The Birth of a Nation*, the racist film produced by two of his academic colleagues from Johns Hopkins University, Thomas Dixon and D.W. Griffith. The film celebrated the KKK as saviors of Aryan culture from the ravages of inferior Blacks.[12]

The conspiracy between Republicans and Democrats to institutionalize racism in America via the Jim Crow system continued through Wilson's administration up through the Truman administration (1945–1953). While the Jim Crow debacle was later reversed through the U.S. Supreme Court's school integration ruling, *Brown v. Board of Education* in 1954 and passage of the U.S. Civil Rights Act of 1964, institutional racism had rooted itself deeply within the United States discriminating against people of color in jobs, education, social security, housing, banking, and virtually all aspects of social and economic portions of American society. While legally dissolved by the U.S. Supreme Court and the Civil Rights Act that ended institutional racism per se, the damage created by the Jim Crow era merely morphed into *systemic racism* and the pervasive, universal biases and prejudices that exist to the present.

Institutional racism was a conscious, yet insidious affair, legitimized by the Wilson administration. Emboldened, the White privileged elite in America saw a political opportunity to manipulate "poor whites" by exploiting racism in the form of Confederate pride. This plan was even endorsed by the U.S. Army, the major agent of policing undesirable minorities—American Indians, African Americans, Asians, and non-White Hispanics. It was during the Wilson years that U.S. Army facilities were named after defeated Confederate officers including those named after the most notorious traitors: Generals Robert E. Lee; Pierre G.T. Beauregard; Henry Benning; Braxton

Bragg; and John Brown Gordon, head of the Georgia KKK. Other Army camps/forts were named after Confederate officers during World War II. Ten U.S. Army facilities are currently named after Confederate officers, including the largest facility in the United States—Fort Bragg in North Carolina. All are in the former Jim Crow South. These facilities were designed as occupational fortresses to remind Black Americans of "their place," especially Black and other minority service personnel throughout the United States as well as emphasizing the relative superior status of "poor whites" vis-à-vis people of color.

Hispanics, notably those of Mexican heritage, suffered the same fate as their Black counterparts in the South. American Indians were not federally recognized as human beings (persons) until Standing Bear's habeas corpus appeal in 1879 and were not considered federal citizens until 1924 when Congress passed the U.S. Indian Citizenship Act. Even then several western states failed to enfranchise Indians residing within their boundaries being forced to do so in the 1970s. Non-White Hispanics, notably those from Mexico or Central and/or South America, are generally considered to be mixed (mestizo) Anglo-Indian or African-Indian. Persecution against "brown Mexicans" has a long history stemming back to Mexico's independence from Spain.

The Texas Rangers, more than any law enforcement or militia, exemplifies the anti-Hispanic/anti-Indian hatred festered in North America from 1821 until 1935. Although portrayed as a heroic force for justice in myth and the media, a closer examination of their history paints a far different picture. Contemporary analysis portrays the Texas Rangers as an extermination squad designed to rid Texas of Hispanics, Mestizos, and American Indians. Texas Rangers trace their origins to 1821 and their law enforcement role among the Austin empresario to protect the former White American settlers from Indian raids in the newly independent Mexico. During the Texas Revolution, the Texas Rangers were expanded into a military-type detachment to range and guard the new Republic. Essentially, they were the Republic's National Guard and could be mustered into the Texas Army as an autonomous battalion. The Texas Rangers were kept somewhat under control during the early years of the Texas Republic under the leadership of Sam Houston, but this changed with the election of Mirabeau Buonaparte Lamar in 1838 whose annihilation policy was to use the Texas Rangers to rid Texas of all Indians through expulsion or massacres.[13]

Following nine years as an independent Republic, Texas joined the United States as a slave state. During the Mexican War, the Texas Rangers served as voluntary irregular cavalry and earned their distinction for brutality. This tradition of brutality continued manifesting itself again during the Mexican Revolution (1911–1917) and the 1915 Plan de San Diego uprising among Hispanics in Texas. The latter was an ill-conceived attempt by a small group of Texas Mexicans (Tejanos) attempting to regain lands lost during the chaos of the Mexican Revolution. U.S. soldiers, who were not permitted by military law to execute prisoners, often turned Mexicans or Tejanos over to local sheriffs or the Texas Rangers knowing that they would execute them without the benefit of a trial. Texas Rangers would leave executed prisoners to rot where they were hanged with empty beer bottles stuck in their mouths. Relatives did not dare to bury their dead with fear of being targeted for death themselves by the sheriff or Texas Rangers.

The Texas Rangers' reign of terror in south Texas led to many Tejanos fleeing across the border never to return. This was the intent of the large Anglo landowners, those who stole the land from the Mexicans in the first place. Robert Kleberg, manager of the King Ranch, advocated for martial law and the internment of Mexicans and Tejanos in concentration camps. Kleberg suggested that when someone was caught, his brothers, half-brothers, and brothers-in-law should also be assumed guilty and immediately arrested or killed.[14] Clearly, the Texas Rangers were to Mexicans, Mestizos, and American Indians what the KKK was to Black Americans until they were brought under the authority of the Texas Department of Public Service in 1935.

The Eisenhower administration (1953–1961) and the conservative Republican Congress initiated Operation Wetback, in violation of the due process dictates of U.S. Constitution. Eisenhower assigned his U.S. Army and West Point colleague, General Joseph (Jumping Joe) Swing, in charge of this illegal operation. Swing was appointed Commissioner of Immigration in 1954 and placed in charge of Operation Wetback where he could conduct his military-type campaign against illegal Mexicans without fear of an international backlash. With the aid of other U.S. Army generals, Swing consolidated the border patrol system into military quadrants where he could muster federal, state, and local law enforcement units in order to sweep up alleged illegals and swiftly deport them without legal recourse. Operation Wetback utilized air-lifts, bus-lifts, train-lifts, and boat-lifts for the purpose of the rapid transportation of captured mojados back to interior Mexico away from the border frontier where they could easily return to the United States. They also introduced the use of tracking dogs in the roundup. Indeed, this multifaceted method of rapid response coupled with quick deportation used another recent military innovation—that of air-to-ground and vehicle-to-vehicle communications, setting the stage for the system still employed by law enforcement today. Anyone of Mexican heritage was stopped and forced to produce proof of their citizenship. Those who could not were part of the roundup regardless of their legal status.[15] The history of Anglo-directed hate and violence toward non-White Hispanics provided the seeds of the current Trump administration's anti-immigration and border wall rhetoric.

In Asia, U.S. intervention extended to the 1850s with America's "gunboat diplomacy" that forced both Japan and China to open their doors to international trade. The 1842 Treaty of Nanking forced China to cede Hong Kong to the British during the *opium war* compelling China to open its doors to the lucrative opium trade. The United States joined Britain in this endeavor with the Treaty of Wanghai two years later effectively setting the date for the beginning of America's massive "drug problem." France and Russia also joined in with the 1858 Treaty of Tientsin resulting in Kowloon added to Britain's China holdings while Russia gained access to portions of Manchuria. Clearly, these forced intrusions into non-White cultures were for the benefit of European and American business enterprises without forethought about the latent consequences of drug trafficking. Another factor relevant to these strong-arm tactics was the influx of not only material trade but the reliance on a cheap labor force for jobs deemed beyond the dignity of White workers.[16]

Chinese males, barred from any hopes of eventual citizenship, immigrated to the United States in the mid-19th century as a source of cheap manual labor in the expanding western states and territories with the first wave arriving during the conclusion of the War with Mexico in 1848 and the doubling of the size of America from land it stole from Mexico. Along with this new addition was the opening of the gold fields of newly acquired California where Chinese coolies (Chinese male laborers) were employed. These same coolies were sought for the dangerous work associated with the construction of the transcontinental railroad. But with the post-Civil War economic woes, Chinese became scapegoats resulting in California passing some of the first discriminatory laws against Asians causing the federal government to take control over racial quotas doing so with passage of the Page Act of 1875. Here, the U.S. government took upon itself the role of classifying Asians as "undesirables." The Page Act was also known as the "Asian Exclusion Act."

What followed was passage of the "Chinese Exclusion Act" of 1882, a move that was endorsed by even the American Medical Association (AMA) stating that Asians, in general and Chinese, in particular, carried germs that were deadly to others. This sounds familiar with the Trump administration attempting to demonize the Chinese for the COVID-19 pandemic of 2020.[17] The "Chinese Exclusion Act of 1882" stayed on the books until World War II when it was repealed in December 1943. Chinese-Americans only gained U.S. citizen status, and 14th Amendment "due process rights," in 1898. Japanese were restricted entry into the United States under the 1907 "Gentlemen's Agreement" with anti-Japanese sentiments peaking in the early years of World War II with President Franklin D. Roosevelt's Executive Order 9066 that authorized the mass incarceration of some 120,000 West Coast Japanese-American citizens. These Japanese-American citizens were forcefully removed from their homes with only the belongings they could carry and placed in stark concentration camps maintained by the U.S. Army.[18]

Weaponizing the judicial system to exclude certain members of society (outsiders) has a long history in the United States where a double standard prevails with laws enacted with the specific purpose of disenfranchising and punishing those designated as out-group members of society—most notably people of color (American Indians, Asian, Blacks, non-Hispanics, etc.), the handicapped, homosexual, or members of non-traditional Christian faiths. A recent judicial ploy designed to exclude Latin Americans and Mexicans seeking asylum in the United States is to criminalize attempted border crossings in the pursuit of this process. Blatant abuses of the adversarial judicial system constitute a form of Kangaroo justice; what the author coins—*Jim Crow Justice*. In essence, Jim Crow Justice is when there are deliberate attempts to rig the system and use illegal and extra-legal processes in order to bring charges and convictions against intended out-group members. Institutionalized racism and the resulting Jim Crow justice system constituted de facto *judicial lynching*—the administration of a double set of legal standards specifically designed to vilify those deemed inferior within society. Studies of judicial lynching extend to early and mid-20th century with research on Blacks in the southern Jim Crow system.

Garfinkel's 11-year, pre-World War II research on judicial biases in North Carolina found a distinctive bias regarding the adjudication of interracial homicides. Blacks killing Whites were considered to be sacred matters with stress placed on getting "the nigger responsible" charged and executed. In contrast, while some White versus White homicides were also considered sacred, this depended on the class of the offender vis-à-vis that of the victim with lower class White offenders prosecuted more aggressively than cases involving Whites of the same class. Secular justice only prevailed when Blacks killed Blacks or Whites killed Whites of their same class.[19] Similarly, Overby, in a review of the administration of justice in the South, noted that many tactics were employed which were deliberately designed to deny Blacks equal justice, including inaccessibility to fair defense counsel, prejudicial prosecution, biased judges and juries, and discriminatory bail practices.[20]

In the United States, this includes African Americans, American Indians, non-White Hispanics, and Asians, while in Europe, with its Aryan elitism, the list of undesirables includes Jews, Serbs, Roma, and non-White immigrants. This process includes rigged juries that exclude members of the defendant's race, ethnic, religious, or social class in order to obtain a conviction, including death penalty cases in the United States. This process evolved in American jurisprudence in the 1970s on the heels of the Civil Rights Movement. A major adaptation to the trial court system, both at the state and federal levels, stemmed from the 1972 *Furman v. Georgia* U.S. Supreme Court case (408 U.S. 238, 345, 1972) that found capital punishment (aka *Death Sentence*) to be in violation of both the 8th and 14th Amendments especially for people of color. Conservative elements in the United States at that time, especially in the South where *Jim Crow* racial discrimination ran rampant for over a century following the U.S. Civil War, fought to reinstate the death penalty, while other developed nations, including Canada, the United Kingdom, and the European Union, discontinued this practice.

In 1976, the U.S. Supreme Court, in response to appeals from Georgia, Texas, and Florida, reinstated the death penalty for states that wished to do so (28 in 2020) with the restriction that it could only be used for first-degree murder convictions. Even then, they had to subscribe to a two-stage process, the first being the finding of guilt of first-degree murder at the jury-trial level, followed by a second phase whereby the same jury would weigh mitigating (life events) versus aggravating (mens rea intent) circumstances prior to a determination of a death sentence. If the mitigating circumstance were seen as being contributing factors, then a life sentence would result in lieu of a death sentence. Within these parameters, the death sentence was reintroduced in 1988 by President Ronald Reagan as part of his Anti-Drug Abuse Act of 1988. Consideration of mitigating circumstances was a major step in viewing individual behaviors within the larger social milieu from which they were socialized whereby acknowledging that individual acts, good or bad, do not occur in a vacuum but rather are contingent upon the social process and environmental bias associated with the collectivity from which the person was raised.

The United States expanded its jurisdictional authority to include quasi-international criminal enterprises in its *War on Drugs* campaign that began with the Richard M. Nixon administration (1969–1974) and continues to the present. In 1970, the U.S. Congress passed the *Racketeer Influenced and Corrupt Organizations* statutes known as RICO. This represented a major revision of the earlier Hobbs Act (Anti-Racketeering Act of 1934) as RICO is a key federal prosecutorial tool in combating drug and related crimes. It departs from the long-held double standard of the U.S. judiciary which puts White-collar crimes in a special category where "cease and desist orders" are issues in lieu of official criminal charges, sparing individuals from criminal liability while allowing the corporate state to be fined without having to admit to any wrongdoing. RICO allowed for criminal intent to be selectively added to the White-collar venue for certain types of crimes. Obviously, RICO is not intended to upset the long-held practice of corporate cheating, graft, and fraud—a powerful political and economic foundation of American Capitalism. Nonetheless, RICO, in its selective administration, allows for individuals (usually Latin American "drug lords") to be criminally charged and their enterprise subject to stiff penalties, property forfeiture, divestiture, and corporate dissolution and reorganization. As stated earlier, the federal death sentence was reintroduced as part of the expanded Anti-Drug Abuse Act of 1988 with the first execution under this provision authorized by President George W. Bush (2001–2009). With the reintroduction of the death penalty, the federal judiciary has deliberately tried death-qualifying cases in states which do not allow capital punishment essentially asserting its bias ostensibly for political effect (conservative vs. liberal agendas).[21]

Given the divisiveness, racism, sectarianism, and political influences within America, the application of judicial ideals are a rarity. The adversarial model does not look for judicial balance as implied but focuses instead on retribution and not reconciliation. Extreme retribution in the United States is the death penalty, and history has shown that it has been disproportionately used against minority populations, notably Blacks, non-White Hispanics, and American Indians. Indeed, the largest official, public execution involved 38 Santee (Dakota) Sioux who were hanged on a single scaffold on December 26, 1862, with President Lincoln's consent. This action followed deliberate provocation by White settlers to starve and enrage the Sioux so that they would again be forced to forfeit lands (ethnic cleansing) for White settlements.[22]

Another blatant example of skewed adversarial justice is the emergence of the *Jim Crow* racism that prevailed in America's South following the "War-between-the-States" (U.S. Civil War), a system that continues to have ramifications in the 21st century. Specifically designed laws were enacted to both disenfranchise and punish Black Americans and other peoples of color. North Carolina, the state with the largest death-row population at the time of *Furman v. Georgia, 1972*, illustrates this travesty of justice. North Carolina was also part of the Cherokee expulsion in 1838. Steiner and Brown, in their book *The North Carolina Chain Gang*, noted that prior to the U.S. Civil War, there were no state prisons and all legal retribution was dispensed at the county (canton) or local level (towns, municipalities). Jails were used only as temporary holding facilities. Following the Civil War, the chain gang emerged as a method of quasi-slavery. Prisoners were placed in enclosed, barred wagons and transported from job to job. Shackles and chains as well as the whip and the sweat box were used as methods of control and added punishment. This form of harsh punishment was mainly for misdemeanor offenses—a sentence that often resulted in death.[23]

Barnes and Teeters referred to the Southern chain gang as "the American Siberia," stating that they were not only discriminatory but manifested some of the cruelest punishment and inhumane treatment ever recorded in American penal history.[24] Blacks made up the vast majority of offenders who were sentenced to the chain gang in North Carolina where, on average, the county chain gang ratio was four Blacks to one White inmate. Prior to the 1972 nationwide death penalty moratorium, the North Carolina death penalty existed for four offenses: first-degree murder, forcible rape, first-degree arson, and first-degree burglary. Most of the death sentences for offenses other than first-degree murder were for Black offenders. A parallel development was the lynching era in the South. According to Ginzburg's book, *100 Years of Lynching*, most lynchings of Blacks occurred following the end of the Civil War and continued until the Civil Rights Movement of the 1960s.[25]

Extra-legal tricks employed by prosecutors include entrapment, agent provocateurs, plea-bargaining witnesses (turning state's evidence), and false charges and planted evidence, devices designed to severely tip the playing field in their favor and against targeted out-groups, most notably minorities of color—Blacks, non-White Hispanics, American Indians, and Asians. Discriminatory justice masquerading as "real" justice has a long history in the illicit drug arena. The discriminatory nature of the *War on Drugs* is often traced to New York governor Nelson Rockefeller and his institution of harsh sentencing for drug-related offenses including mere possession for one's personal use. These laws, known as *The Rockefeller Drug Laws*, established mandatory minimum sentences of 15 years to life for possession of four ounces of narcotics, a sentence similar to that for second-degree murder. These laws set the stage for harsher penalties across the nation leading to America having the largest incarcerated population of any developed nation.

The problem with the drug laws was that while the majority of persons using or selling drugs are White, the harsh consequences of these laws were directed at African Americans and Hispanics. The vast majority of Blacks and non-White Hispanics received the severest prison terms, while White offenders often received more lenient sentences throughout the country in both state and federal jurisdictions. Convictions for "crack cocaine," used primarily by the less affluent and minorities, received far harsher sentences than for "powder cocaine" used by the affluent, notably Whites, even when the amounts were equal. The difference between minority and White justice is illustrated by the fact that there is a double set of laws where if White commits the offense, it is processed as a misdemeanor, while people of color, and poor Whites, are charged with a felony for the same offense leading to a disproportionate number, in both raw numbers and per capita, of Blacks, American Indians, and non-White Hispanics with a record of felony convictions.

Felons have been disenfranchised in many states and in federal jurisdictions until recent court challenges. As of 2013, 11 states denied felons the right to vote eliminating up to 10% of the state's Black population from voting. Changes are being sought during the "Black Lives Matter" campaign that addresses the high incident of unarmed Blacks being executed by White police officers. Changes to these blatant, racially based, injustices are slowly coming about. New York's laws were reformed in 2004 under Governor George Pataki, while, at the federal level, Congress passed a law in 2010 substantially lowering recommended sentences for those convicted of crack cocaine crimes. In June 2012, the U.S. Sentencing Commission made these new laws retroactive for those sentenced prior to these changes, a move that will affect some 12,000 federal prisoners. While efforts are currently underway to change this injustice, some White conservative states are attempting to further delay felon's voting rights by imposing stiff fines and then making them ineligible to vote until they pay off these improbable fines. Furthermore, four conservative states, three in the old Jim Crow states (Arkansas, Georgia, South Carolina) and Wyoming, still have not enacted "hate crime statutes" despite the national trend of other states and the federal government.

The public pressure to attempt to correct historical injustices toward poor and minority drug users does not extend to the so-called drug lords. This has led to a federal effort to capture more international, Latin American drug cartel leaders. While this media campaign scores political capital for the administration, it seldom has any lasting effect given that the demand for these illicit agents is as strong as ever. Arrest under the Foreign Narcotics Kingpin Designation Act involves a funding scheme whereby the United States pays local Mexican, Central American, and South American officials for the arrest and deportation of cartel leaders. In order to do this, lower level cartel members, usually the most dangerous ones, are paid to "turn state's evidence." These "plea-bargain witnesses" are offered immunity or reduced charges in return for offering evidence that will justify the apprehension and extradition to the United States of the cartel's higher echelon. Oscar Martinez wrote of how this process operated in Central America in his book, *A History of Violence*:

> "There was a regional summit here (Guatemala) and Secretary of State Clinton came down. She said that for every $3 we put in [in the fight against drug trafficking] they would put in $1. It's a bad joke, because in the end we're putting money that we could have used for education, health, many other things." The arrest of the Guatemalan barons isn't anything more than fear of the sword hanging over the state's head. It's more survival than it is strategy. The battle against drug trafficking in Guatemala is not a decision grounded in sovereign agency. It is a battle they are thrust into.[26]

The race-based justice in the United States is evident in the current opioid crisis that has taken tens-of-thousands lives changing the drug user's profile from racial minorities to Whites. Now monies are being poured into treatment and prevention, while those accountable for this crisis, the big pharmaceutical companies, are given a pass—this despite clear evidence of premeditation on the parts of corporate leaders. Again, it's the double standard of justice: one set of rules for minorities—harsh penalties and incarceration; and yet another set of rules for White-collar criminals—fines and "cease and desist orders" without the stigma of culpability.

In 2020, the COVID-19 pandemic further complicated matters by focusing on the deadly consequences of institutional racism in America with a disproportionate death rate among people of color, notably African Americans, American Indians, and non-White Hispanics. It was during the pandemic that worldwide attentions were again galvanized on the "Black Lives Matters" movement focusing on the killings of Black males at the hands of White police officer. The 2020 episodes began with the stalking and killing of Ahmaud Arbery, who was jogging in a White Georgia neighborhood on February 23 where he was pursued by White vigilantes and shot to death. Next followed the May 25 widely distributed video of the murder of George Floyd, a handcuffed, unarmed, Black male chocked to death by a White police officer in Minneapolis. And, again in Georgia, a widely distributed video captured the scene of a White police officer shooting Rayshard Brooks in the back as he was fleeing detention on June 12. All three men were of African American descent. These incidents rekindled the "Black Lives Matters" protest, not only in the United States but worldwide calling for real changes within law enforcement but also calling for a reassessment of institutional racism within American society.

Social Justice and Legal Ethics

Social justice is an important component of restorative justice in that it looks at how societies treat their members. It addresses formal (manifest/de jure) and informal (latent/de facto) processes that determine the preferred social hierarchy (social stratification). This process determines the relationship between in-groups versus out-groups. The social order, in turn, is determined by rules that articulate the "dynamics of inclusion" (in-groups) versus the "dynamics of exclusion" (out-groups). Race, class, age, gender, social economic status, and sectarianism are dynamics of stratification and relevant factors to be considered in any viable analysis of restorative justice.

Social justice analysis falls into two basic categories—*distributive* and *procedural* justice. Distributive justice addresses how the society and its members view the "fairness" of the allocation (distribution) of what it defines as scarce resources. This falls mainly within the realm of *de facto justice*. Procedural justice, on the other hand, looks at the formal rules (laws, statutes, customs, etc.) that dictate how these resources are allocated. For the most part, this process falls under *de jure justice*. *Social justice* addresses the difference between procedural and distributive justice. Hence, policies that establish the rules that set the standards for the implementation of criminal, civil, and family/juvenile justice fall into the category of procedural justice. Criminal, civil, and family/juvenile justice adjudication, on the other hand, fall on a continuum with restorative justice on one pole and retributive justice on the other. That said, it is important to remember that regardless of the extent of written or customary traditions, the administration of justice, per se, is a human process and in that sense we need to recognize the psychological processes that influence how individuals, or groups, perceive the fair allocation of justice. Institutional racism is when society adopts a double standard of justice while, at the same time, pretending that its judicial ideals and procedures are equitable and fair. Jim Crow justice and legal lynching are examples of institutional racism in America exemplifying the long tradition of preserving the powers of the White elite.

The American Psychological Association was one of the first major international professional organizations to not only address America's double standard of justice, it made recommendations to Congressional leaders for immediate changes on June 16, 2020:

> On behalf of the 121,000 members and affiliates of the American Psychological Association (APA), I am writing to express our great appreciation for your leadership in addressing racial disparities by holding the U.S. Senate Judiciary Committee hearing tomorrow on Police Use of Force and Community Relations. Our nation is in the midst of a racism pandemic, and it is past time to fix these inequities by making bold reforms in our policing laws and practices. APA believes longstanding change starts with our willingness to acknowledge racism as a public health crisis, as well as our openness to engage in honest dialogues about our criminal justice system. Racism has dire consequences, particularly for our African American citizens and other communities of color, who disproportionately suffer from the structural inequities and personal biases embedded within our society. Since the 1940s, psychologists have made fundamental contributions to our understanding of the nature of prejudice, stereotypes, and their impact on shaping human actions, emotions, and judgments. It is from this scientific evidence-base that we submit our congressional testimony for your consideration, which includes the following recommendations:
>
> - Promote community policing. APA calls on Congress to implement community-based policing nationwide. Research shows that this approach increases community trust.
> - Ban chokeholds and strangleholds. These tactics can be deadly or have serious neurocognitive impacts. These solutions should account for the safety of the officer in dangerous situations, as well as the safety of individuals interacting with law enforcement.

- Invest in crisis intervention teams. Psychologists play a key role in community-based, crisis intervention teams that train police officers to safely and effectively deal with situations involving individuals with serious mental illness. Tailored by each community to fit local needs, these teams unite the efforts of police officers, mental health educators, and community advocates to resolve and de-escalate potentially violent situations in positive ways.
- Increase the number of mental health professionals in law enforcement agencies. Mental health professionals can provide training and resources to help identify and defuse potential conflicts between law enforcement and the community. They are also skilled in identifying and addressing issues affecting police officers and staff including stress, trauma, family support, and education.
- Involve psychologists in multidisciplinary teams to implement police reforms. These professionals need to be empowered to help monitor police officers' stress levels, mental health, burnout, and attitudes toward the public. Police psychologists are needed to help optimize police department cultures, develop leaders, and institute a "preservation of life" policing orientation.
- Encourage private/public partnerships between mental health organizations and local law enforcement. These partnerships can develop best practices for addressing community and police relations that can be disseminated widely across the nation to police departments and mental health facilities. Police-community partnerships encouraged by the Community Oriented Policing Office (COPS) of the Department of Justice (e.g., athletic leagues) can decrease stereotypes and increase citizen engagement.
- Discourage police management policies and practices that can trigger implicit and explicit biases. Research shows that certain types of proactive policies may be more effective at reducing racial disparities than are interventions designed to eliminate implicit bias.
- Strengthen data collection. Created following recommendations by the Task Force on 21st Century Policing, the Police Data Initiative supports local police department efforts to leverage data to increase transparency and accountability and build trust with their communities. Different from data on crime, these datasets may include data on stops and searches, uses of force, officer involved shootings, or other police actions.
- Bolster research. APA calls for re-establishing a Science Advisory Board at the Department of Justice to help bridge the divide between research and practice in criminal justice fields.

Through regular interactions with the Office of Justice Programs leadership and staff, members of the board would gain a deeper appreciation of the complexities of implementing and evaluating innovative approaches to the administration of criminal and juvenile justice. APA stands ready to assist the Judiciary Committee in finding impactful bipartisan solutions to address racial disparities and improve trust in our policing systems.

Sincerely, Arthur C. Evans, Jr., PhD Chief Executive Officer.[27]

Notes

1 Benton-Cohen, K. 2018. *Inventing the Immigration Problem: The Dillingham Commission and Its Legacy.* Cambridge, MA: Harvard University Press.

2 *Ibid.*

3 Terman, L.M. 1916. *The Measurement of Intelligence.* Boston, MA: Houghton Mifflin.

4 *Buck v. Bell,* 274 U.S. 200, 205, No. 292 United States Supreme Court, 1927.
5 Op. cit. 7, p. 26.
6 Barnes, H.E., & N.K. Teeters. 1959. *New Horizons in Criminology* (3rd ed.). Englewood Cliffs, NJ: Prentice-Hall, Inc.
7 Black, E. 2003. *War against the Weak: Eugenics and America's Campaign to Create a Master Race.* New York, NY: Four Walls Eight Windows.
8 Becker, H.S. 1963. *Outsiders.* London, England: The Free Press.
9 ACLU. 2020. *The Constitution of the United States of America.* Washington, DC: American Civil Liberties Union, pp. 28–29. www.aclu.org.
10 *Plessy v. Ferguson,* 163. U.S. 537 (May 18, 1896).
11 French, L.A. 2018. *The History of Policing America. From Militias and Military to the Law Enforcement of Today.* Lanham, MD: Rowman & Littlefield.
12 *Ibid.*
13 Gwynne, S.C. 2010. *Empire of the Summer Moon: Quanah Parker and the Rise and Fall of the Comanches, the Most Powerful Indian Tribe in American History.* New York, NY: Scribne.
14 Johnson, B.H. 2003. *Revolution in Texas: How a Forgotten Rebellion and Its Bloody Suppression Turned Mexicans into Americans.* New Haven, CT: Yale University Press.
15 Garcia, J.R. 1980. *Operation Wetback: The Mass Deportation of Mexican Undocumented Workers in 1954.* Westport, CT: Greenwood Press.
16 French, L.A., & Manzanarez, M. 2019. *Borders and Immigration: The Geo-Politics of Marketplace Demands and Ethnic Relations.* Lanham, MD: Lexington Books.
17 Op. cit. 11.
18 *Ibid.*
19 Garfield, H. 1949. Research Note in Inter- and Intra-Racial Homicides. *Social Forces,* Vol. 27, pp. 381–396.
20 Overby, A. 1972. Discrimination in the Administration of Justice. *Race, Crime and Justice* (Reasons, C.E., & Kuykendall, J.L., eds.). Pacific Palisades, CA: Goodyear Publishing Company, pp. 264–276.
21 Op. cit. 16.
22 French, L.A. 2007. *Legislating Indian Country: Significant Milestones in Transforming Tribalism.* New York, NY: Peter Lang, p. 56.
23 Steiner, J., & Brown, R.M. 1927. *The North Carolina Chain Gang.* Chapel Hill, NC: University of North Carolina Press.
24 Op. cit. 6.
25 Ginzburg, R. 1962. *100 Years of Lynching,* New York, NY: Lancer Book.
26 Martinez, O. 2016. *A History of Violence: Living and Dying in Central America.* London, England: Verso.
27 Evans, A.C. 2020. American Psychological Association's June 16th racial justice recommendations addressed to U.S. Senators Lindsey Graham and Diane Feinstein.

3

INFORMED CONSENT

Informed consent refers to the agreements without hidden agendas, coercion, fear of retaliation, or deceit. It also alludes to the social-educational, emotional, and psychological maturity of the individual involved. In most instances, an age ceiling is required by law making it an offense for someone taking advantage of those considered to be "minors." Another major variable in addition to the age/maturity/competency issue is that of how people are classified and stratified within human groups. Caste and class played a major role in some of America's most notorious cases of human exploitation by seemingly "ethical" institutions such as academia, the medical profession, and federal agencies. Here, institutional racism and White elitism often act in concert in conducting clandestine "medical research" purportedly for the "greater good." The Tuskegee experimentation on economically impoverished and ill-educated African American men from 1932 to 1972 exemplifies a sad chapter in America's exploitation of what it considered a lower racial caste within the United States.

The Tuskegee Syphilis Study

The Tuskegee Syphilis Study is important in that its disclosure in 1972 exposed a long-hidden truth about America's racist past and the corresponding mechanisms of institutional racism embedded throughout government and professions, notably the medical profession, that served to promote White supremacy and a privileged elite. The Tuskegee study also predates that world's reactions to these atrocities following the end of the World War II (WWII). Even then, the United States was able to conceal its own clandestine medical atrocities for another 30 years. Not only did America's dominance in the WWII ad hoc International Military Tribunals (IMTs) help it draw attention from its own medical atrocities, its "victor bias" allowed it to "mine" the data from both German and Japanese medical experiments while downplaying the human rights significance of these medical atrocities.

The Tuskegee Syphilis Study is rooted in the eugenics era in which the United States played a major role providing a model for other societies including that of Hitler's Nazi regime. The eugenics movement in the United States was endorsed at the highest levels of academia, the medical profession, and government. It emerged during the resurgence of the racial caste system

DOI: 10.4324/9781003224426-3

known as "Jim Crow" whose growth exploded following President Wilson's endorsement during his administration. White supremacy and Jim Crow segregation were opposite sides of the same coin. Eugenics was yet another tool for legitimizing and furthering "institutional racism" in America. Indeed, during the Jim Crow/eugenics era, Confederate dominance was manifested by the proliferation of monuments, statues, plaques, schools, roads, military bases, buildings, parks, and other visible reminders of White supremacy while reinforcing the inferiority and subjugation of people-of-color (Blacks, American Indians, Asians, non-White Hispanics) issues only being adequately addressed in mid-2020 following a series of killings (modern lynchings) of unarmed, often handcuffed, Blacks at the hands of White police officers leading to the resurgence of the "Black Lives Matter" (BLM) movement.

The clandestine use of lower class Black subjects for dangerous biomedical experiments like the Tuskegee Syphilis Study occurred during a time of planned "demographic genocide" whereby poor Black, American Indian women, and others so-called inferior breeders, were secretly sterilized as part of the American eugenics program. These programs operated without the knowledge or consent of the victim yet were justified under the prevailing "science" of the day. This process involved psychological testing in order to determine the genetic inferiority of the "feeble minded" within society. Here, eugenics and racism are closely intertwined providing a seemingly objective rationale for social discrimination under the guise of "intellectual testing."

American Eugenics Movement

The flaw in this thinking was that the parameters for testing human suitability were designed by the privileged White elite within American society. Toward this end, they developed a classification system for determining those who are socially unacceptable, a process that became part of the medical lexicon for over a century despite changing the original terms, *idiot*, *imbecile*, and *morcn* with three levels of mental retardation: mild, moderate, and profound—all based on intelligence tests originally designed to weed out the socially inferior from American society. The founding fathers of "science-based eugenics" were two noted psychologists—Lewis M. Terman and Robert M. Yerkes. Both served terms as president of the prestigious American Psychological Association (APA), Terman in 1923 and Yerkes in 1917.

Terman, a professor at Stanford University, was influenced by his mentor, Francis Galton who was considered to be the founder of "scientific psychology" setting the stage for so-called objective measures designed to determine a human classification continuum relevant to "Social Dawinism."[1] The foundation of psychological testing was seen as the predictive factor in determining social suitability, a critical factor in the selection of involuntary sterilization designed to cleanse society of its undesirables allowing for a superior human gene pool. Lewis Terman provided the measurement for determining mental suitability with his adaptation of the 1908 French Binet–Simon mental assessment tool.

Terman flaunted his 1916 *Stanford-Binet test* as an objective eugenic measure in determining those of inferior human status suitable for either lifelong institutionalization or forced sterilization or both. The main problem was the test's reliability and validity in that was normed using the upper-class White faculty and families at Stanford University, one of the most elite educational institutions in America. Nonetheless, Terman promoted his test as an objective measure, one that reinforced the privileged White elite at the expense of others in American society.[2]

Terman's work coincided with both President Wilson's endorsement of segregation and the advent of amassing an army to fight in the World War I (WWI), a process that involved assessing draftees from different races, ethnic groups, and social economic strata, including those from the Jim

Crow South. What was needed was an intellectual assessment tool that could measure the draftee's suitability for service while, at the same time, discerning between those who were English literate and those who were illiterate. This task was assigned to the APA which comprised a Committee on the Psychological Examination of Recruits. It was chaired by the APA president, Robert Yerkes, along with Lewis Terman.

This effort resulted in the development of two alternative tests, one for literate recruits (Army Alpha) and one for those deemed English illiterate (Army Beta). Both used the new *Intelligence Quotient* (IQ) metric utilizing the "ratio IQ" format (which later relied on a deviation IQ format where a normal IQ was based on a norm of 100 with two standard deviations about norm). The APA described this new method of assessing military fitness as follows:

> The purpose of psychological testing are (a) to aid in segregating the mental incompetent, (b) to classify men according to their mental capacity, (c) to assist in selecting competent men for responsible positions ... The success of this work in a large series of observations, some five thousand officers and eighty thousand men, make it reasonably certain that similar results may be expected if the system be extended to include the entire enlisted and drafted personnel and all newly appointed officers.[3]

Given that these tests only measured one's verbal IQ, that is the extent of someone's educational status, it served to reinforce the marked social divides at the time especially in the grossly inadequate school system provided for the poor and minority communities in America at the time. It was not until 1939 and the introduction of the *performance IQ* subtests that a more realistic measure of general intelligence could be ascertained. The Wechsler–Bellevue test and subsequent adaptations measured both the verbal (level of education) and performance IQ (raw intelligence) leading to a general IQ based on both these subtests. This led to the new Army General Classification Test (GCT) used during the WWII and up through the Vietnam War.

The main issue is that psychological testing was used mainly to reinforce the privileged position of White supremacy and the inferiority of others. Testing was seen as a scientific justification of eugenics and the dynamics of exclusion in American society for over a century—from the post-Civil War era to the Civil Rights era of the 1960s and 1970s. The basic argument put forth was that testing provided scientific evidence as to the inferiority of minorities and poor Whites given that they scored well below their better educated, higher class counterparts. A major flaw in this argument is that these early IQ tests only measured "verbal IQ" which was biased by using the educational standards of the privileged White elite. Accordingly, both Terman and Yerkes, in particular, and psychologists, in general, were held in high regards by the White privileged elite at the time in that they shared the prevailing eugenic philosophy with the Carnegie Institution, Rockefeller Foundation, Harriman Rails, Kellogg, Harvard, and other elite universities, and even the Smithsonian Institution, the National Geographic Society, and the U.S. Bureau of Ethnology which was documenting America's indigenous cultures.[4]

The road to building America's superrace in the early decades of the 20th century saw an increased popularity in both the Ku Klux Klan (KKK) and the eugenics movement. So strong was the eugenics movement and its effort to purify American society that by 1926, 23 states enacted compulsory sterilization laws which the U.S. Supreme Court condoned in its ruling, *Buck v. Bell*.[5] Forced sterilization was widely practiced among Blacks and American Indians, often without their knowledge or consent, during the Jim Crow era by both state and the federal governments up until the 1970s and the time of the Tuskegee Syphilis Study's disclosure and termination. Even the Nazi abuses of the eugenics movement did not fully curtail its practices in America.

Clearly, the sanctioning of eugenics and its basic thesis of White supremacy served to embolden institutional racism and the legitimatization of segregation in all aspects of American society resulting in discrimination in all facets of society creating a self-perpetuating, self-fulfilling prophecy of White superiority and minority inferiority. The harsh reality of this mind state was that it legitimized violence in the form of vigilantism, riots, lynchings, even massacres, as well as condoning police abuse and killing of minority suspects. It provided the foundation for the overincarceration of non-Whites in America's prisons and jails via the institutionalized "double-standard of justice," issues only seriously being assessed in 2020 in the resurgence of the BLM movement.[6]

As mentioned earlier, not even the Nazi atrocities committed under the guise of eugenics and ethnic cleansing was cause for America's elite to adequately reevaluate its own institutional racism. It became apparent that America did not want to have its own system of race/ethnic and class structure opened to worldwide scrutiny following the end of the WWII and the subsequent IMTs. Indeed, America set the stage for, and dominated, the ad hoc IMTs—both the Nuremberg Tribunal for Germany and the International Military Tribunal for the Far East (IMTFE) for Japan—ostensibly for two reasons: firstly, to conceal America's own eugenic experiments like the Tuskegee Syphilis Study; and, secondly, to glean insights into the Nazi and Japanese human experiments for American adaptation.

The human subject medical abuses were kept separate from the images displayed at the trials held in Nuremberg, Germany. Instead, the "Medical Case" involving 20 doctors and 3 medical assistants (Case No. 1), along with 11 other cases, were prosecuted in the United States outside the limelight or international participation of the main trials. These "Subsequent Proceedings" were held from October 25, 1946, through April 1949. They were adjudicated by U.S. civilian judges presiding over military tribunals with each tribunal consisting of a bench of three or more judges who were admitted to serve temporary terms of five years. Case No. VIII, the Race and Resettlement Case, also had relevance to the ongoing Tuskegee project and Jim Crow segregation and America's sordid history of ethnic cleansing directed toward American Indians, in that it would have focused on America's long history of institutional racism. By hiding these proceedings from the public, the United States was cleverly able to keep its own eugenic practices and illegal human subject experiments concealed from scrutiny.[7] A similar process occurred at the IMTFE proceedings that convened on April 29, 1946. General Douglas MacArthur virtually dictated the conditions of the IMTFE focusing on so-called Class A offenses, crimes committed by Japan's top wartime leaders, with the exception of the Emperor. Conspicuously absent from the public trials were the human subject experiments and Unit 731's open-air tests of germ warfare on civilians. Again, this was a planned omission from the public record and only emerged decades later in 1981 in an article by John W. Powell published in the *Bulletin of the Atomic Scientists.*[8]

The Tuskegee Syphilis Study addressed both the impact of American eugenics and the extent of institutional racism in the United States in that it used a convenient lower-caste racial subset in order to find a solution to a pressing medical issue at the time—the long-term effects of syphilis. The problem was that deceit was employed from the onset of the study from its early days during the Great Depression. A larger ethical problem beyond the issue of "informed consent" was the seemingly sadistic continuation of the study after a cure was found for syphilis and the fact that the poor Black subjects were denied access to this treatment. The issue of institutional racism was the complicity between the government and medical elites. The project only came to light 40 years following its inception in 1932 in an expose written by Jean Heller of the Associated Press that surfaced in 1972. This was the same time that federal and state forced sterilization programs, condoned by the U.S. Supreme Court in 1932, were also exposed and subsequently ended. Clearly, the forced sterilization of lower class minorities, notably Blacks and American Indians, was more widespread, and like the Tuskegee Syphilis Study, involved deceit.[9]

A sad commentary regarding both of these programs is that they persisted years after the U.S. Supreme Court ended the Jim Crow era they ordained in 1896 in *Plessy v. Ferguson* with their 1954 *Brown v. Board of Education* decision condemning racial segregation and its accompanying policies of racial exploitation.[10] Equally appalling is that both of these programs were endorsed by the U.S. Public Health Service (PHS), the quasi-military federal organization that uses Navy rank for its officers; the same organization that provides Indian Health Service (IHS) for enrolled member of *Indian Country*. Unquestionably, many of the clandestine sterilizations of Indian women occurred in IHS hospitals—the only medical facilities available to most tribal residents supposedly protected as federally dependent wards of the U.S. government.

Adding to the eugenics movement was the slave-era stereotype of the content slave, genetically endowed to serve White masters. Mixing ideology and medical science, American physician, Samuel A. Cartwright, offered a clinical/biological explanation for "runaway madness"—a disease afflicting some Black slaves—which he termed, *drapetomania*. Cartwright cited the Bible and its call for slaves to be submissive to their master seeing this symbiotic relationship as God's will for human harmony:

> If treated kindly, well fed and clothed, with fuel enough to keep a small fire burning all night—separated into families, each family having its own house—not permitted to run about at night to visit their neighbors, to receive visits or use intoxicating liquors, and not overworked or exposed to too much to the weather, they are very easily governed—more so than any other people in the world. If any one or more of them, at any time, are inclined to raise their heads to a level with their master or overseer, humanity and their own good requires that they should be punished until they fall into that submissive state which was intended for them to occupy. They have only to be kept in that state, and treated like children to prevent and cure them from running away.[11]

Cartwright saw the malady of "runaway madness" as a problem stemming from Whites who try to treat slaves as equals. The doctor even offered some examples for premorbid behavioral risk factors found in slaves with a predisposition for running away: sulky and dissatisfied without cause. The corresponding treatment prescribed for this malady was a severe whipping as a preventive measure while the amputation of the slave's big toes would prevent them from running away. Published during the enactment of The Fugitive Slave Act by the U.S. Congress on September 18, 1850, Doctor Cartwright's thesis resonated well in the South fueling the intrusion of bounty hunters through the free states during the turbulent decade preceding the U.S. Civil War (War between the States). Cartwright's thesis provided another argument for the Confederacy's succession beyond the U.S. Constitution's 1793 (Article IV, Section 2) denying slaves "due process" hence allowing federal judges to decide the fate of alleged fugitive slaves.[12] While the Civil War ended slavery as a legal institution in the United States (13th Amendment; Abolition of slavery) in 1865, the Jim Crow era facilitated a de facto form of servitude and the institution of a rigid caste system, one that was given a formal stamp of approval with the 1896 U.S. Supreme Court, *Plessy v. Ferguson*, decision and resurgence racial-biased eugenics movement emboldened during the decades leading to the WWII.

This was the setting for the Tuskegee Syphilis Study. Blacks were, with few exceptions, considered certifiably inferior to Whites and therefore not eligible for civil rights protections, such as due process, allowing the medical profession to use them with impunity as experimental subjects. The Tuskegee study's initial six-month project has morphed into four decades making it the longest nontherapeutic human subject project in medical history. The project gained its legitimacy under the auspices of the U.S. PHS. Unlike most medical research where the efficacy of a drug or procedure is not only time limited but conducted under experimental designs that involve "double-blind" control versus experimental samples. The Tuskegee study, *The United States Public Health Service Study of Untreated Syphilis in the Negro Male in Macon County, Alabama*, although not initially designed as such, ended up being a longitudinal study without any preventive measures to treat its subjects. To further shroud it from public scrutiny, the study was housed at the U.S. Center for Disease in Atlanta, Georgia.[13]

The Tuskegee Syphilis Study incorporated the inherent racial biases of the eugenics era, notably that Blacks differed significantly from Whites both mentally and physically. In this sense, the study was not designed to benefit mankind per se but to medically demonstrate the nature and extent of the inferiority of Blacks. The study was based on the premise that Blacks were neurologically inferior to Whites and therefore only suffered the physiological effects of devastating diseases such as syphilis and cardiovascular problems. This racial bias led to gross neglect during the four decades of the study, including denying the Black subjects access to treatment with the penicillin once it was discovered to be a cure for venereal diseases (VDs); the use of barbaric techniques incorporated in the study; and abuse of the bodies of the 128 men who died during the study. Add "deceit" to this list in that the Black male participants and their spouses and children were told that the study was designed to study effects of "bad blood" and not that their participation in the program was to medically torture them resulting in a death sentence for some. In essence, poor, uneducated Blacks, from the Jim Crow South, were used as higher-functioning lab animals.

A sad commentary on the Tuskegee Syphilis Study is the complicity of faculty and staff at the Tuskegee Institute (now Tuskegee University), a noted Historical Black College/University (HBCU) that emerged during the Jim Crow era to provide teachers and medical personnel to service the Black population during segregation. The Tuskegee Institute was a preemptive HBCU founded by Booker T. Washington. The affiliated hospital, along with other HBCU medical facilities, was enticed by the U.S. PHS to let its medical facilities, including staff, be used for the study. Although the PHS researchers and administrators were White, retrospective analysis of the involvement of Tuskegee-trained Black medical personnel shows that their participation in the study was crucial for its continuation. While it is easy to place special blame on a Black HBCU for its involvement in the Tuskegee Syphilis Study, it is important to keep in mind that the country, indeed, much of the world, at the time the program was initiated, was in a deep economic depression.

The Depression afflicted Black institutions more than others, including higher education making it difficult not to take advantage of support from the highest levels of the federal government, notably the U.S. Surgeon General. The bane of this criticism is Eunice Rivers, a Black nurse who effectively managed the Black subjects for the four-decade duration of the study. We are learning more about the complicated role institutional racism plays on society as a whole. A major finding of the *Brown v. Board of Education* 1954 U.S. Supreme Court decision that legally ended Jim Crow segregation was the results presented by Black psychologists, Drs. Kenneth and Mamie Clark, who showed the prevalence of institutional racism and the mass socialization of White supremacy with their "doll study" whereby both White and Black children, given the choice of race-appropriate dolls, overwhelmingly selected the "White doll."[14]

Within this scheme, a hierarchy of power is clearly established where a person is taught not to question his/her superiors. This is especially the case within both the military and the medical profession. An associated feature of both institutional racism and White supremacy is that of "entitlement" which has its own stratification. Those at the top are the most entitled with certain professions mandating universal compliance. This represents "manifest entitlement" like that associated with people in authority. Latent entitlement, on the other hand, refers to an inherent acknowledgment of one's privileges. In the Tuskegee experiment, doctors had a higher level of entitlement than nurses, while White medical professionals held higher levels of entitlement than their Black counterparts. Accordingly, in order to keep her job, nurse Rivers followed the protocol expected of her—that of passive obedience, following the doctor's orders.[15]

Deceit was not the only troubling aspect of the Tuskegee experiments, unnecessary crude, often cruel methods were employed on these unwitting subjects much like the experiments by Germany and Japan conducted on prisoners of war (POWs) during WWII. One reason for America's experiments on poor Blacks was the prevailing belief that the subjects were sub-humans more akin to animals than their White counterparts. These abuses including subjecting them to painful and dangerous spinal taps and denying treatment even after the discovery of penicillin in blatant violation of the 1943 Henderson Act that required both testing and treatment for VD. Of the 600 Black male samples, 399 were positive for late-stage syphilis. These men, and affected members of their families, suffered tumors, blindness, heart disease, paralysis, and mental illnesses, and when they died, their bodies were dissected for further study under conditions that one of the leading doctors termed "necropsy"—that used to describe animal autopsies.[16]

The Tuskegee experiment was not the only one used to study VDs during this time era where the government was anxious to curb the spread of VD among American GIs (military personnel). In addition to the Southern Black sharecropper sample, other studies were designed as well including a Guatemala sample. Again using a non-White sample. (Guatemala had a population that is mostly Indigenous Mayan Indians). The fight to curb the spread of VD, notably syphilis and gonorrhea among GIs, led researchers to another venue—that of Guatemala. Drs John F. Mahoney and John Charles Cutler of the U.S. PHS Venereal Disease Research Laboratory first tried enticing federal prisoners as paid subjects for their research but within a year found their study to be nonproductive concluding that sexual intercourse was a missing ingredient within this population. Cutler then fostered a relationship with a Guatemalan doctor, Juan Funes, to begin the study in Guatemala, where not only was prostitution legal but the country had a low rate of VD in comparison to the United States. Thus, he began the Guatemala VD experiment from 1946 to 1948.

The intent of the study was to test the efficacy of different medications in combating the rate and extent of VD infections. With the consent of the Guatemalan government, the U.S. medical researchers had access to the military, mental hospitals, orphanages, and prisons. As part of the study, psychiatric female patients were inflicted with syphilis. Another component of the study was to unwittingly infect female prostitutes and then entice them to have sex with multiple men in a row with neither partner aware of the designs of the research. In all, some 5,500 Guatemalan prostitutes, soldiers, prisoners, children, and psychiatric patients unwittingly participated in the two-year study with about a quarter deliberately infected with VD without their consent. Law suits were subsequently filed against Johns Hopkins University, the Rockefeller Foundation, and Bristol-Myers Squibb Pharmaceuticals. U.S. President Barack Obama apologized to Guatemalan President, Alvaro Colon, for the United States' involvement in these studies in October 2010.[17]

Prisoners: Cheaper Than Chimpanzees

The use of prisoners as unwitting subjects for medical experiments was highlighted by Jessica Mitford in 1973 following shortly after the expose on the Tuskegee Study. Mitford noted that using prisoners for medical experiments was cheaper than using chimpanzees. She also noted the link between these clandestine experiments and those conducted by German doctors during WWII claiming that the Nazi doctors cited these as part of their defense:

> In their defense the accused doctors cited comparable experiments carried out on prisoners by American physicians: in 1906, a group of Philippine convicts were given "an abundance of cigarettes and also cigars if they desired them" for submitting to infection with plague and induction of beriberi ... In 1915, pellagra was induced in 12 Mississippi convicts, all of whom became seriously ill. They were rewarded by the promise of early parole. In 1944, several hundred Illinois and New Jersey prisoners were infected with malaria so that new cures could be tried out on them. They were paid in dollars. Some became extremely ill with malaria, others suffered horribly from the toxic effects of the experimental "cures."[18]

Following the Nuremberg trials, efforts were made worldwide to curb the use of prisoners in dangerous medical experiments due to the fact that while they may "consent" to the experiments, they seldom are made aware of the dangerousness involved to their person. And in many instances, deceit is a common practice and, certainly, they are easily subject to coercive influences. Mitford noted that in 1961, the international efforts to prohibit the use of prisoners as subjects led to the World Medical Association proposing that, "being captive groups, they should not be used as the subjects of experiments." The resolution was never implemented due to the strong opposition by American doctors.[19]

A major stimulus for using prisoners, other than being cheaper than chimpanzees, was the lucrative pharmaceutical industry and their need to follow Federal Drug Administration (FDA) regulations requiring that all new drugs had to involve human trials. This process involved three stages. In Phase I, the new drug needed to be tried relevant to its effectiveness and possible toxic properties, and then it moved on to Phase II, whereby a substantial sample of healthy humans are administered the drug in order to determine the therapeutic limits of safety for the agent. If the new agent passes both of these phases, it is given as medication to patients in order to test its efficacy as a remedy for the cited illness. This phase generally involves the use of a double-blind study between an experimental sample (those administered the agent) and a control sample given a placebo. The advent of new medications following WWII led to a rush to market these agents worldwide and lobbying clout contribution to not only "informed consent" but to the issues of "duty to disclose."[20]

COVID and College Consent Contracting

The most basic meaning for "informed consent" is the subject's legal consent to participate in a program or project that is clearly defined including any potential aftereffects. This process involves a full disclosure of the program's intent and design as well as an understanding of the participant's mental and legal capacity to make an informed consent absent of promised enticements or punishments associated with their participation. For an "informed consent" to be legal, the individual needs to be of legal age and sound mental status in order to make this judgment. Informed consent goes beyond medial research and includes consent to a number of therapeutic venues and other research endeavors. In the fall of 2020, in a controversial move, colleges and universities are proposing having students, faculty, and staff sign consent agreements exonerating the institution of liability from contacting COVID-19 while on campus or involved in institutional activities. This may be problematic for students whose legal status is that of a minor, therefore requiring the formal consent from their legal guardian, the actual holder of privileges. The protocol at the University of New Hampshire system is offered as an example:

> Informed Consent Agreement for Students Participating in On-campus Programming for the Fall Semester The University of New Hampshire (UNH) is looking forward to welcoming students, faculty and staff back to our campuses for in-person instruction. We will need the help, cooperation and participation of you and every other member of our university community to maintain a reasonably healthy and safe environment. While none of us can ensure each campus will be free from the risk of contracting COVID-19, by working together we can manage and mitigate the risk. We ask you to help reduce the risk of transmission by staying current on information about the virus provided by public health officials and experts. UNH has established and implemented public university-wide protocols COVID-19 website page designed to limit the spread of COVID-19 on its campuses and to help safeguard vulnerable persons on its campuses, in the Town of Durham, in the cities of Manchester and Concord, and in the wider community for the 2020–21 academic year. Stay Informed UNH has been following the directives of the governor of the state of New Hampshire, the U.S. Centers for Disease Control and Prevention (CDC), and New Hampshire's Department of Health and Human Services (DHHS) to guide us in our approach to delivering our curriculum to our students and opening our campuses for the fall semester. We refer you to our COVID-19 website page to reference useful and important public health resources and the school's prior communications on this topic. You may also access the Governor of State of New Hampshire CDC's website—New Hampshire's DHHS website Commitment to Health and Safety UNH is developing protocols and policies for students' learning and activities both on and off of its campuses. These protocols and policies will include guidelines for students, faculty and staff to support UNH's efforts to maintain a safe and healthy campus environment, and will include: Wearing Masks or cloth face coverings—while in class, and in public common areas, community members will be required to wear a cloth face covering. Physical Distancing—while wearing a mask, maintain six feet between you and others when possible. Gatherings—according to NH DHHS guidance, avoid social gatherings involving large groups of people. Hand Washing or Sanitizing—frequently throughout the day • Immunization—students will be subject to UNH Health and Wellness immunization protocols • Pre-Arrival Testing—all students, faculty and staff will be required to show proof of a negative COVID-19 test result before arriving for the fall semester COVID-19 website page. Additional Testing—all students, faculty and staff will be subject to periodic COVID-19 testing COVID-19 website page. Temperature screening—as established by NH DHHS, students, faculty and staff may be subject to temperature screening protocols. Contact Tracing—all students, faculty and staff will be subject to contact tracing protocols COVID-19 website page. Symptom Monitoring and Reporting—all students, faculty and staff will be expected to self-monitor their health and report any COVID-19 symptoms or exposure to individuals with COVID-19 or its symptoms to UNH Health & Wellness. Isolation and Quarantine—students, faculty and staff who test positive for COVID-19, are symptomatic or were in contact with those who test positive for COVID-19 may be subject to isolation and quarantine protocols. Waivers—students may be required to execute waivers of liability if they desire to participate in certain extracurricular activities or in order to attend certain events or functions.
>
> Download and activate any required UNH approved public health applications It is important that we work together to follow protocols, policies and guidelines that are

established by UNH. Our protocols will be updated from time to time based on evolving guidance and directives from the State of New Hampshire and the CDC. We will notify you of these updates and will post them on our website. Failure to adhere to these protocols will be considered a violation of the Code of Conduct included in the Student Rights, Rules and Responsibilities and may result in discipline, to include removal from campuses.

If You Feel Sick If you experience any COVID-19 symptoms (listed below), we may require you to be tested, remain quarantined until the test results are available, and, in the event of a positive test, remain in isolation until cleared by a health care professional for return to in-person classes and other on-campus activities. Students may be asked to return home if that is possible. UNH is establishing isolation and quarantine facilities on or near the Durham campus that will include access to online versions of your educational programs, food, and access to health care as needed. According to the CDC, COVID-19 symptoms include (but may not be limited to): Fever or chills, Cough, Shortness of breath or difficulty breathing, Fatigue, Muscle or body aches, Headache, New loss of taste or smell, Sore throat, Congestion or runny nose, Nausea or vomiting, Diarrhea.

Tuition Obligations Regardless of the learning environment for fall 2020, UNH tuition will be the same. The tuition you pay is in exchange for learning, academic credit, and certain non-academic services that will be provided whether in person, in a hybrid environment, or entirely remotely. Please Read Carefully Before Signing: By signing below, I understand the University of New Hampshire's approach to on-campus learning during the COVID-19 pandemic. I understand that my decision to return to on-campus programming is voluntary. I understand that UNH cannot guarantee my health or immunity from infection. I understand there are risks of exposure to the virus from symptomatic and asymptomatic carriers. I recognize that the risks of exposure to COVID-19 include sharing space with others and engaging in interpersonal communications. I assume the risks associated with being at the University of New Hampshire including the risk of exposure to COVID-19.

I affirm my obligation to cooperate in making the campus reasonably safe, and consent to attending all university activities.

Yes, I agree to the terms to be on campus. ______________________________
________ __________________ Signature of Student

Date ____ Print Name ___________
______________________________ ______________________ Signature of Parent/
Guardian (if student under age 18) Date ______________________________
____

Print Name No, I do not agree and wish to take all classes online _______________
__________________________ ______________________ Signature of Student

Date ____ Print Name _________
______________________________ ______________________ Signature of
Parent/Guardian (if student under age 18) Date ___________________________
_________ Print Name.[21]

The APA, under the section on Human Relations, provides a model template for consent from which most clinical associations follow:

> 3.10 Informed Consent (a) When psychologists conduct research or provide assessment, therapy, counseling, or consulting services in person or via electronic transmission or other forms of communication, they obtain the informed consent of the individual or individuals

using language that is reasonably understandable to that person or persons except when conducting such activities without consent is mandated by law or governmental regulation or as otherwise provided in this Ethics Code. (See also Standards 8.02, Informed Consent to Research; 9.03, Informed Consent in Assessments; and 10.01, Informed Consent to Therapy.) (b) For persons who are legally incapable of giving informed consent, psychologists nevertheless (1) provide an appropriate explanation, (2) seek the individual's assent, (3) consider such persons' preferences and best interests, and (4) obtain appropriate permission from a legally authorized person, if such substitute consent is permitted or required by law. When consent by a legally authorized person is not permitted or required by law, psychologists take reasonable steps to protect the individual's rights and welfare. (c) When psychological services are court ordered or otherwise mandated, psychologists inform the individual of the nature of the anticipated services, including whether the services are court ordered or mandated and any limits of confidentiality, before proceeding. (d) Psychologists appropriately document written or oral consent, permission, and assent. (See also Standards 8.02, Informed Consent to Research; 9.03, Informed Consent in Assessments; and 10.01, Informed Consent to Therapy.[22]

Notes

1 Galton, F. 1869. *Hereditary Genius: An Inquiry into Its Laws and Consequences.* London, England: Macmillan.
2 Terman, L.M. 1916. *The Measurement of Intelligence.* Boston, MA: Houghton Mifflin, p. 26.
3 Thorndike, R.M., & Lohman, D.F. 1990. *A Century of Ability Testing.* Chicago, IL: The Riverside Publishing Company, p. 44.
4 French, L.A., & Manzanarez, M. 2019. *Borders and Immigration: The Geopolitics of Marketplace Demands and Ethnic Relations.* Lanham, MD: Lexington Books.
5 *Buck v. Bell,* 274 U.S. 200, 205, No. 292, U.S. Supreme Court, 1927.
6 Black, E. 2003. *War Against the Weak: Eugenics and America's Campaign to Create a Master Race.* New York, NY: Four Walls Eight Windows Press.
7 Spitz, V. 2005. *Doctors from Hell: The Horrific Account of Nazi Experiments on Humans.* Boulder, CO: Sentient Publications.
8 Powell, J.W. 1981. A Hidden Chapter in History. *Bulletin of the Atomic Scientists,* (October), pp. 44–52.
9 Reverby, S.M. (ed.). 2000. *Tuskegee's Truths: Rethinking the Tuskegee Syphilis Study.* Chapel Hill, NC: University of North Carolina Press.
10 See *Plessy v. Ferguson* (163 U.S. 537, 1896) and *Brown v. Board of Education* (347 U.S. 483, 1954).
11 Cartwright, S.A. 1851. Report on the Diseases and Physical Peculiarities of the Negro Race. *The New Orleans Medical and Surgical Journal,* (May), pp. 691–715.
12 *Ibid.*
13 CDC, *Syphilis Study at Tuskegee: The Tuskegee Timeline.* Washington, DC: The Center for Disease Control and Prevention, U.S. Public Health Service. www.cdc.gov/tuskegee/timeline.htm.
14 Clark, K.B. 1967. *Dark Ghetto: Dilemma of Social Power.* Middletown, CT: Wesleyan University Press.
15 Jones, J. 1981. *Bad Blood: The Tuskegee Syphilis Experiment.* New York, NY: Free Press.
16 *Ibid.*
17 Rodriguez, M.A., & Garcia, R. 2013. First, Do No Harm: The U.S. Sexually Transmitted Disease Experiments in Guatemala. *American Journal of Public Health,* Vol. 103 (12), pp. 2122–2126.
18 Mitford, J. 1973. *Kind & Unusual Punishment: The Prison Business.* New York, NY: Alfred A. Knopf, pp. 138–139.
19 *Ibid.*
20 Reiter, K. 2009. Experimentation on Prisoners: Persistent Dilemmas in Rights and Regulations, *California Law Review,* Vol. 97, pp. 501–566.
21 See *www.unh.edu.*
22 See APA *Ethical Principles of Psychologists and Code of Conduct.* www.APA.org.

4

DUTY TO DISCLOSE

Regulating Advances in Medicine

Related to the "Informed Consent" is the duty to disclose. With the advent of rapid advances in pharmacology beginning in the late 1950s, drugs were seen as a panacea for a host of physical and mental afflictions. Indeed, the use of Thorazine (chlorpromazine) and Lithonate (lithium carbonate) led to the discovery of numerous other agents that eventually led to the feasibility for home and community care, a phenomenon that ended the process of live-long institutional care and the emptying of mental hospitals worldwide. The problem was that potentially dangerous side effects were not adequately investigated prior to marketing certain of these drugs leading to devastating effects. A more serious issue was the concealment of potentially dangerous side effect by pharmacological manufactures in order to rapidly market their products. The marketing of the drug thalidomide illustrated this issue.

Thalidomide was developed and marketed in the late 1950s as a nonbarbiturate sedative at a time when alarms were raised concerning the addition properties of anxiolytics, and hypnotics like Valium (diazepam) and Librium (chlordiazepoxide) were also developed and promoted at this time. Thalidomide was advertised as being completely safe for everyone, even pregnant mothers. By 1960, the drug was sold in 46 countries for its intended purpose. An Australian obstetrician, however, discovered that thalidomide also alleviated morning sickness among pregnant clients and thus began its "off-label" (application of agent for purposes other than for which the drug was approved/intended) use for pregnant mother. The severe birth defects associated with its use, notably children born with phocomelia—a condition resulting in shortened, absent, or flipper-like limbs—was quickly noted in 1961, and the drug was soon banned in Germany and by 1962 by most countries.

Fortunately, the U.S. Federal Drug Administration (FDA) inspector, Francis O. Kelsey, was instrumental in preventing thalidomide's approval in the United States despite pressure from the powerful pharmaceutical firms and others. Kelsey was adamant that the data were inadequate and did not meet the safety required for a drug's approval for general use in America, doing so at a time when clinical trials were not required for FDA approval. The ensuing debacle in countries using thalidomide off-label for morning sickness led to passage in 1962 of the Kefauver-Harris Drug Amendment Act.[1]

DOI: 10.4324/9781003224426-4

The Kefauver-Harris Act (PL 87-781) actually served to strengthen the existing Food, Drug, and Cosmetic (FD&C) Act of 1938 stating that for drug needed to be proven safe before they gained federal approval for marketing: a requirement that led to the need for human trials. This amendment required that drug manufacturers to provide proof of the effectiveness and safety of their product for it to meet with FDA approval for marketing. The safety component included accurate information concerning "side effects" such as those associated with thalidomide when used off-label. The 1962 Amendment also prohibited drug companies from preventing their agents from entering the less expensive generic drug market by slight modifications or renaming their product merely to maintain a higher cost to customers.[2]

PL 87-781 articulated the scientific process needed for FDA approval, including the use of humans in clinical trials. No longer could drug companies merely present their "data" relevant to the agent's safety. Now, the "safety" issue would be determined by the New Drug Application (NDA) process which eventually led to the guidelines spelled out by the Investigative New Drug (IND) process that called for adequate and well-controlled studies which included the following or a combination of these control protocols:

1. A clear statement of the objectives of the study along with the research design and trial results;
2. The research design needs to be a quasi-experimental design that compares an experimental sample with that of a control sample; and
3. The research design needs to articulate the particulars of the study including sample size, duration, and statistical measures allowing for independent replication. Five types of controls are allowed:
   (a) Placebo concurrent control where subjects are randomly assigned to either the experimental or control group;
   (b) Dose comparison concurrent control where subjects are assigned to one of several dose level of the treatment;
   (c) No treatment concurrent control where subjects are assigned to a treatment or no-treatment sample;
   (d) Active treatment concurrent control whereby subjects are either assigned to the experimental drug or an existing agent that has already been approved for the treatment of the medical condition for which the new agent is being tested for without knowing which is active and which is a placebo; and
   (e) Historical control where subjects are assigned to the proposed treatment only with their responses compared with those of similar subjects not in the trial.[3]

In addition to the duty to disclose potential adverse drug reaction, informed consent was also required for subjects employed in the clinical trial component, a factor that apparently was not retroactive to either the Tuskegee Study or the forced sterilization programs that continued for another decade following passage of the Kefauver-Harris Drug Amendments.

The Sampling Dilemma: Students, Prisoners, and Veterans

Human subject research, especially that involving medical and/or medical experiments, have had a difficult time finding adequate subjects especially since the exposes of the 1970s and the restrictions demanded by the FDA. Colleges and universities have long used their undergraduate students as subjects for nonmedical experiments, some with serious psychological consequences. Among faculty researchers are notable psychologist whose studies raised serious questions concerning the psychological welfare of their student subjects. Stanley Milgram's, *Obedience to Authority* and Philip Zimbardo's *Stanford Prison Experiment,* both conducted in the early 1970s, became classic examples of the unanticipated psychological consequences of short, seemingly harmless studies using students. Timothy F. Leary, a Harvard psychology professor, involved students and prisoners in his psychedelic therapy studies using psilocybin hallucinogenic mushrooms and, later, lysergic acid diethylamide (LSD). The major issue that emerged from these and similar studies was any notification that the subjects could withdraw when feeling distressed by the experiment. This led to the added criterion to any human subject study's "informed consent" protocol—they now had to be notified in advance of the experiment that they could withdraw at any time without suffering any negative consequences, such as a lower grade or suspension from the school or their program of study. Another condition was the provision of aftercare counseling and therapy for any unanticipated conditions, mental or physical resulting from these experiments.[4]

Subsequently, the notoriety of these studies, especially given the exposes of the Tuskegee and the civil rights and anti-war social unrest at the time, led to demands for better protection of students from the exploitation of faculty eager to engage them in their research resulting in the creation of Human Subject Research Institutional Review Boards (IRBs). Currently, every public and private institutions of higher education require an IRB for any project involving human subjects, notably "students." Research hospitals and neuropsychiatric facilities added bioethics committees in order to review research and procedures, especially when consent was not a sufficient safeguard.

Few realized at the time that the Stanford Prison Study was a federally initiated project funded by the U.S. Office of Naval Research. Given that it was now more difficult to use students acting as prisoners, a movement to again use real prisoners was renewed by researchers at home and abroad. Federal funding for university research has a long history in the United States. In addition to the Tuskegee study by the U.S. Public Health Service, the U.S. Atomic Energy Commission (AEC) funded postwar research in the 1950s of radioactive iodine on the health effects on newborn babies and pregnant women in conjunction with the University of Iowa and the University of Nebraska College of Medicine. Other human radiation AEC experiments were conducted up through the 1970s in Nashville, Cincinnati, Chicago, and Boston all without informed consent or warnings as to the potential harmful effects of these clandestine studies. Added to this mix were the Central Intelligence Agency (CIA) LSD experiments of the 1950s where unsuspecting American civilians were given the drug as a part of the U.S. Chemical and Biological Warfare program.[5]

Increased focus on both informed consent and the duty to disclose the exact nature of the research design, including potential lasting effects, essentially limited the college student pool for serious and challenging research notably those involving clinical trials. Hence, the focus was again on using other captured audiences, prisoners, and military veterans. Americans, Canadians, and European researchers have recently called for the use of prisoners in their clinical trials. In the United States, a federal panel of medical advisors from the National Academy of Sciences and the Institute of Medicine recommended the loosening of government restrictions regarding the use of clinical drug trials using prisoners, both those incarcerated and those out on parole or probation, effectively freeing up a potential sample of some 7 million subjects.[6]

Medical researchers noted that prior to the exposes of the 1970s, like that of the Tuskegee study, about 90% of all pharmaceutical products were tested on prison inmates. Nonetheless, oversight still remains a major obstacle given that in 2,000 several universities were cited for their use of federal monies for conducting research on prisoners while failing to provide detailed findings from their experiments. While the use of prisoners for medical and drug experiments saw a dramatic decrease in Europe following the World War II, there has been a resurgence from medical researchers to reintroduce this practice. Opponents maintain that a major problem is attempting to generalize prisoner results to the larger general population especially in countries that do not come close to America's proportion of incarceration. Accordingly, the United Kingdom's National Research Ethics Service, the agency that approves clinical trials involving National Health Service patients, maintains that research among prisoners should relate directly to their health care, a position similar to Canada.[7]

Military veterans have been used as experimental subjects while both on active-duty status and as discharged veterans under the care of the U.S. Veterans Administration. Active-duty military personnel, including federally activated Army and Air Force National Guard members, fall under the auspices of the U.S. Department of Defense (DOD), while those who already served come under the care of the U.S. Department of Veterans Affairs (VA). Both groups comprise a vast pool as research subjects. Indeed, many medical innovations came about during combat situations which, on the one hand, saved many lives, while, on the other hand, rendered many service personnel disabled. In order to adequately address the needs of this growing population, arrangements have been forged between teaching medical hospitals and military and VA hospitals.

From the Civil War era to the Great Depression, a collection of federal, state, and private entities took care of disabled veterans. On July 21, 1930, President Herbert Hoover signed Executive Order S. 398 creating the Veterans Health Services and Research Administration with the mandate of supervising the collections of 54 hospitals at that time serving 4.7 million veterans mainly from the Spanish American War and the World War I. The first VA administrator was Brigadier General Frank T. Hines whose tenure extended to the end of the World War II in 1945. The end of the World War II added an addition 16 million veterans to the 4 million World War I veteran pool. Added to this burden was the popular 1944 GI Bill that provided education and training for veterans. The Korean Conflict and Vietnam War added to the demands placed upon the VA. While conscription ended in 1973 with the new "all-volunteer force," the demands for military personnel during the Persian Gulf War added federalized National Guard troops into the mix, including, for the first time, a substantial number of females.

Just prior to the onset of the Persian Gulf War, in 1988, the U.S. Congress passed Public Law 100-527; the Department of Veterans Affairs Act elevating the VA to a cabinet-level federal agency. While signed by President Ronald Reagan on October 25, 1988, it actually became effective on March 15, 1989, under President George H.W. Bush. The VA is one of the largest federal agencies whose mandate includes the Veterans Health Administration (VHA) component and the vast array of VA hospitals and clinics as well as research on female veterans' health needs, military sexual trauma (MST), post-traumatic stress disorder (PTSD), suicide, and traumatic brain injuries (TBIs); the Veterans Benefits Administration (VBA) component that deals with home loans, disability claim, retirement benefits, and GI Bill funding; as well as the National Cemetery Administration which is responsible for all veterans cemeteries except Arlington National Cemetery which remains under the U.S. Department of the Army. Since 1982, the U.S. Congress added a fourth mission to the VA, that of aiding in civilian crisis situations working with both the Federal Emergency Management Agency (FEMA) and/or the Department of Health and Human Services (HHS). The latter is a vital tool in the 2020 COVID-19 response plan. Unfortunately, these increased demands for veteran health care led to critical delays in care at VA hospitals, some resulting in untimely deaths. An expose in 2014 uncovered the widespread practice of VA administrators' falsification of wait-time for appointments in order to cover up the inadequacies of providing timely and needed care to veterans, leading to the resignation of Eric Shinseki, the Secretary of VA on May 30, 2014.[8]

Case Study: The Boston VA Valproate Acid Experiment

The author enlisted in the United States Marine Corps (USMC) in February 1959 when I was 17 and still in high school (four-months deferred entry). I served four-year active duty with the Second and Third Marine Divisions earning the Navy/Marine Expeditionary Medal for Cuba (1961) and the Armed Forces Expeditionary Medal for service in Southeast Asia (1963). I served his remaining reserve time in Manchester, New Hampshire, and later in Hawaii when I was in the process of being reactivated. During my physical in Hawaii, a federal psychologist processed me for disability-related injuries sustained during my active duty. Hence, I was awarded a disability compensation in late 1964, administered intelligence and aptitude tests, and was found eligible for the college track under the original GI Bill. Subsequently, in February 1965 following my honorable discharge, I matriculated at Church College of Hawaii (now the Hawaii campus of Brigham Young University) beginning my academic career that resulted in an undergraduate degree, two masters, and two doctorates (PhDs).

The disability and educational benefits were administered under the old consolidated Veterans Administration of 1930 and its subsequent additions during and following the World War II. The VA essentially provided myself, and others like me, with lifelong, affordable health care. The GI Bill training component, however, depended upon the motivation and abilities of the individual veteran. Influenced by the Japanese-American VA psychologist who processed me in 1964, I pursued degrees in sociology and psychology, eventually earning doctorates in both fields, disciplines that require substantial research training. Even then and while working in state neuropsychiatric facilities as a staff psychologist, I was not sufficiently aware of the VA's human subject research process. That is, until I unwittingly became a participant in a major research project—the valproate acid trials conducted at the Boston Veterans Administration Hospital in May 1989—two months following the elevation of the Veterans Administration to the cabinet level along with the newly created position of Secretary of VA.

My involvement was due to the onset of major motor (grand mal) seizures following an attack by a neurologically impaired, dangerous client at one of the New Hampshire Neuropsychiatric facilities. My involvement in the valproate acid trials provided me with a unique ethnomethodological (participant observer) experience relevant to the nature and extent of veterans used as human subjects in clinical trials. Although enrolled in the state's Blue Cross/Blue Shield insurance pool, I continued to use the VA facilities for major health issues such as the dizziness and subsequent Grand Mal seizures. Not only was the VA now under a single federal cabinet-level authorization, new medical technologies were emerging as well as a newly revised diagnostic classification of mental disorders—the *Diagnostic and Statistical Manual on Mental Disorders* (*DSM-III*). By the time the *DSM-III* arrived on the scene in 1980, a new classification was added to the anxiety disorders—that of PTSD a syndrome afflicting a substantial proportion of Vietnam-era veterans. This and underreported TBIs were seen by some as being the underlying cause for the marked increase in veteran's suicides at the time—a number that was matching the total in-county U.S. deaths of over 58,000 veterans. Unfortunately, the VA was attempting to conceal another devastating effect of the Vietnam war—that of the effects of Agent Orange.

While the state had access to Dartmouth Medical School personnel and equipment, the VA had the latest technological devices, including that of computerized tomography—the computerized tomography (CT) scan. At the time of the onset of the assault (May 9, 1989) and subsequent seizures (May 11, 1989), the itinerate CT-scan trailer was at the Manchester VA facility. This is when my initial scan was performed. The results indicated a chronic subdural hematoma which resulted in my being sent to the larger Boston VA hospital that had the other new device of the time allowing for a magnetic resonance image (MRI) of the suspected brain infarct. (The medical scientists who discovered the CT and MRI were subsequently awarded the Nobel Prize in Medicine for their work.) Unbeknownst to me, the Veterans Administration was involved in a major neurological study designed to determine if valproate acid (Depakote) was more effective than the currently used medication, Tegretol (carbamazine) in regulating not only seizures but impulse control disorders secondary to TBIs. Having to be hospitalized in order to ascertain the exact nature of my subdural infarct, I was assigned to their clinical trial whereby each of us involved (all current or former enlisted personnel—no officers). We were then locked into our ward on the seventh floor of the VA research hospital for 10 days (May 24–June 2, 1989).

As I found out later, this was a double-blind study where neither the main neurologist, Dr. Thomas R. Browne, M.D., nor the clinical trial subjects (myself included) did not know if we were assigned to the experimental group (those administered the active ingredient—Depakote and a Tegretol placebo) or to the control group (those administered active Tegretol and a Depakote placebo). Only a third-person nurse practitioner knew the group assignments. Surprisingly, we were confined to the "neurological ward" and not allowed to leave for the 10-day confinement period. We were issued special brown hospital gowns and apprehended if we attempted to leave. I asked about this given that clients on the "psychiatric ward" were giving free movement of the facility and was told that they are not potential dangerous clients while we were. What was hidden on the seventh neurological floor were significantly impaired veterans suffering from serious side effects of Agent Orange exposure. In retrospect, I realized that this may have been a major reason to consolidate VA facilities during the Reagan administration—that is to conceal the seriousness of neurological damage secondary to Agent Orange. Those of us who were ambulatory finally could leave following the daily tests and observations by a host of doctors from surrounding teaching hospitals. Many others were actually incarcerated in the secure neurological ward with little treatment choices. One veteran pleaded with me to assist him in his suicide attempt. This was a profound ethical challenge given my training in psychology versus my compassion for a suffering veteran.

Once released, we were assigned to other VA facilities so that our medication regiment could be traced and reported to Doctor Brown's group. Thus, for 18 months, we continued to take the combination of active and placebo medications and had our blood work drawn on a regular basis. Two months following the hospitalization component, I was in New Mexico at my new job at Western New Mexico University where I was assigned to a doctor at the Silver City VA outreach clinic and further monitored by the large VA medical facility in Albuquerque and its affiliate—the University of New Mexico Medical School. I was shocked to learn that I was required pay for the medicine administered during the trial and afterwards. Moreover, there was no explanation provided as to the ethology of my prefrontal lobe injury, one that obviously dated back to my Marine Corps tours. Adding insult to injury, the VA denied my claim for compensation consideration relevant to the seizures stating that the medical records kept by the USMC were too vague at the time of my deployments especially concerning head injuries. A comment among veterans under VA care at the time was that Mrs. Reagan was telling us to say "no" to drugs while her husband, the President, telling the VA to say "no" to Agent Orange, PTSD, and TBI claims. This duplicity led me to pursue additional postdoctoral training in the area of neurophysiology and neuropsychology leading to my eventual unilateral termination of the Depakote doing so during the summer of 1996 fortunately without any reoccurrence of seizure activity.

This experience brought up two major concerns, informed consent and duty to disclose.

Apparently, I agreed to participate in the study if only to receive the necessary treatment for my seizures, which frightened me at the time, and while I keep meticulous records, I could find no written "consent to participate" in my files. There certainly is no record of the detailed testing and results which were never provided despite my numerous inquiries for my own records relevant to the 18-month study. Despite being trained as a psychologist at the prestigious Burros Institute at the University of Nebraska, many of the medical tests were unknown to me such as CT scan, MRI, positron emission tomography (PET) scan, brain electric activity map (BEAM), Holter monitor, glucose tolerance tests, electroencephalography (EEG), etc. More importantly, I do not recall being given the opportunity to withdraw from the study or to be provided with a drug with fewer severe side effects. The VA's "carrot and the stick" technique was that either you participated or else chanced losing your benefits.

Although regular blood work was required, what was not disclosed was Depakote's potential for liver damage, especially at the high levels used to control seizures and impulse control disorders. The discomfort associated with my Depakote regiment, gas, weight gain, hair loss, dietary restrictions, and the potential for a compromised liver motivated me to take advanced studies in the area of neuropsychology where the conventional wisdom at the time was that the maximum time for effective neuro-compensation, that is dendrite repair surrounding neural damage such as my prefrontal subdural hematoma, was seven years. Given that I had followed the prescribed drug regiment for seven years, I unilaterally slowly titrated my Depakote during the summer of 1996 without any rebound seizure activity. I then notified my VA primary care doctor of my actions. Fortunately, while concerned about a rebound effect, he ultimately concurred with my action and the rationale for discontinuing my medication. Not knowing the other subjects in my experimental cohort, I could not share my experience with others.

The Opioid and Coronavirus Crises and Their Antecedents

Government oversight relevant to informed consent and the duty to disclose potential harmful effects stemming from human subject research, as specified by the 1962 Kefauver-Harris Amendment to the 1938 Federal FD&C Act, has again been challenged with the current opioid and COVID-19 crises. While the opioid crisis emerged prior to the 2020 coronavirus pandemic, the two influenced each other as social stressors worsened during the COVID-19 pandemic. A primary issue in both situations is the role that drugs play in these situations. Notably, milestones in substance enhancement and in psychopharmacology changed the methods of treatment within the United States and Western societies beginning with the advent of anti-psychotic agents in the 1950s with Thorazine and other neuroleptics followed by the introductions of benzodiazepines as treatment for alcoholism (Valium, Librium, Klonopin, Ativan, Xanax, BuSpar, Neurontin, etc.) and the use of hypnotics & psycho-stimulants for relaxation and/or stimulation (Halcion, Ambien, Benadryl, etc.).

A new wave of medications entered the scene in the 1980s with the selective serotonin reuptake inhibitors (SSRIs): Prozac (fluoxetine), Zoloft (sertraline), Paxil (paroxetine), Celexa (citalopram), etc. Although designed as treatment of anxiety and depression, they soon became personal-enhancement agents like methylphenidates and cocaine. The development and marketing of new-grade pain medications such as OxyContin and fentanyl, promoted as being nonaddictive by its manufacturers, contributed greatly to the current worldwide drug crisis. This plus the increased use of heroin and "meth" added to the recreational and self-medication markets already in play. What distinguishes the United States from other cultures is that it allows drug companies to advertise their products widely, including on television. This, coupled with little or no federal oversight and a strong political lobbying effort, has contributed to skyrocketing cost increases even for basic medications, contributing to a health-care crisis even before the advent of the coronavirus pandemic. Clearly, the opioid crisis brought a new focus on both drug enforcement and treatment considerations given the widespread nature of the population involved. No longer could drug abuse be seen as only a problem afflicting lower class, people of color in America.

Substance use/abuse is often rooted in the cultural milieu and one's with acknowledgment that individual variations such as potential for addiction also needs to be factored in. Dr. Clay Rivers wrote of the cultural variations in his 1994 book:*Alcohol and Human Behavior:Theory, Research, and Practice*. Rivers noted that cultures that used alcohol under controlled circumstances usually had the lowest rates of alcoholism. This included European Jews, French, and Italians—those cultures where drink was associated with positive social events such as meals and social and religious rituals, whereas societies that prohibited alcohol (Methodists, Baptists, Mormons, etc.) had the highest rate of substance abuse by those who did use alcohol.[9] America's substance-use dilemma extends to its earliest days. W.J. Rorabaugh's book, *The Alcoholic Republic:An American Tradition*, notes that between 1790 and 1840, Americans drank more alcoholic beverages—nearly a half pint of hard liquor per man each day then at any other time in our history. He noted:

> Alcohol was pervasive in the first fifty years of the Republic. Men were taught to drink as children-even babies, though women were by no means faint-hearted abstainers ... they drank because they thought liquor was healthful and nutritious ... because whiskey was superior to bitter beer, sour wine, muddy water ... And of course Americans also drank for the sake of getting drunk.[10]

Popular medical cures often mixed alcohol with other substances such as opium and/or cocaine. A call for temperance emerged due to a number of factors including massive public intoxication and the pursuit of a *moral imperative*. Indeed, the United States' "*War on Drugs (substances)*" began early in the Republic's history with the Whiskey Rebellion (1791–1794).

The "moral imperative" emerged as a reaction to the Catholic and Jewish mass immigration of the middle and late 19th century where Protestantism was associated with abstinence and temperance as an indication of their moral superiority, leading to passage of the 18th Amendment to the U.S. Constitution (prohibition of liquor) in 1919 and its eventual Repeal (21st Amendment) in 1933. Clearly, Prohibition represented a strong sectarian and ethnic bias a trend that continued to dominate the United States' *War on Drug.*

In support of this thesis, the two most elitist and influential groups during and following the Revolution, the conservative Puritans of New England and the slave holders of Virginia, both once endorsed alcohol drinks. Both Increase Mather and his son, Cotton Mather, preached that "drink was a good creature of God," while President Thomas Jefferson is credited with inventing the "presidential cocktail party. *s.*[11]"The U.S. involvement in the drug crisis began when it joined the Opium Wars when China banned the opium trade in 1799, a lucrative capitalist trade for Great Britain (France, Russia). Great Britain declared war on China in 1839 with the United States joining the Opium Wars in 1844 using its *gun boat diplomacy.* The United States also used this as a means of exporting cheap Chinese laborers to build the transnational railroad. But racism in the United States soon turned these same drugs used to open China to Western markets to discriminate against foreign immigrants, notably the Chinese. This long history of racial discrimination began in the late 19th century with the Chinese Exclusion Act (1882) eventually leading to the Harrison Narcotic Act of 1914 which used taxation as a tool for outlawing opium and heroin.[12]

Two U.S. agency directors, Harry J. Anslinger and J. Edgar Hoover, in their respective roles as Director of the Federal Bureau of Narcotics (forerunner of Drug Enforcement Agency [DEA]) and the Federal Bureau of Investigation (FBI), were instrumental in instituting the race bias basis for the ensuing contemporary *U.S. War on Drugs (substances)*, starting early in the 20th century. U.S. federal enforcement agencies emerged in 1920 in response to Prohibition with the Federal Bureau of Narcotics established in 1930 providing Director Anslinger his *reefer madness* pulpit culminating in passage of the 1937 Marijuana Transfer Tax Act that augmented the 1914 Harrison Narcotic Act to include marijuana, a substance popular among Blacks, Hispanics, and American Indians and other impoverished groups in America.[13]

J. Edgar Hoover, a close colleague of Anslinger, used the FBI to discriminate against U.S. minority populations of color. Their joint efforts lasted over 30 years into the turbulent 1960s and 1979s resulting in the criminalization of drug use and the marked increase of incarceration of minorities in local and federal penal facilities. The Anslinger/Hoover "race drug criminal profile" continues to the present. The DEA emerged from the Federal Bureau of Narcotics under the Nixon Administration (1969–1974) with his formal declaration on the *War on Drugs* and passage of the Racketeer Influenced and Corrupt Organizations Statutes (RICO). But it was President Ronald Reagan (1981–1989) who militarized the DEAs by involving the FBI, CIA, and the U.S. military in international antidrug operations. President Reagan reintroduced the Federal Death Penalty as part of *the Anti-Drug Abuse Act of 1988*. It was designed to execute convicted "drug kingpins." The current Trump Administration's Attorney General (Barr) gave notice in July 2019 that the United States will again start executing federal prisoners beginning in the fall. Clearly, the so-called *War on Drugs* is responsible for both the increased militarization of law enforcement in the United States as well as the disproportionate incarceration of people of color.[14]

Currently, the United States is undergoing an epic drug crisis—one that crosses racial, ethnic, and socioeconomic/class divides giving new emphasis on prevention and treatment and not just focusing on the criminalization of users and dealers. The drug death rate is the leading cause of death (64,000+ in 2016) surpassing mortality due to human immunodeficiency virus, auto crashes, or firearms (which is the highest for any developed nation). The nature of the current drug crisis adds a new social/clinical dimension to the existing legal structure forcing a national review of both big pharmacology business practices and America's "pain free" perspective—a correlate of the massive media blitz of drug manufactures offering "cures" for most aliments real or imagined.

The dilemma for the United States is its race-based double standard for dealing with the drug crisis. On the one hand, it wants to continue to deal harshly with members of minority groups while, on the other hand, promote "mental health" alternatives for the "White" addicts. Criminalize minority users/dealers while offering treatment options for Whites. This double standard of justice also extends to the adjudication of "white-collar" versus "black market" drug pushers. This schizophrenic trend sees President Trump advocating executing "drug dealers" like they do in the Philippines while, at the same time, allocating more resources for treatment and preventive efforts. While Joaquin Guzman aka "El Chapo," head of the Sinaloa Mexico drug cartel receives a life term without parole in the U.S. "Super Max" prison, The Sackler family, head of Purdue Pharma, whose drugs OxyContin, etc. are linked to nearly 49,000 overdose deaths, get to pay fines and stay out of prison.

The opioid crisis forced law makers to reassess past measures that tended to punish low-income and minority drug users while offering White offenders treatment paths to recovery. Methadone has long been used in the treatment of opium addictions while benzodiazepines were once popular with alcohol treatments. More recent additions, such as buprenorphines (Naloxone, Narcan nasal spray, Evxio, Suboxane, etc.)—opioid antagonists—have played a significant role in current drug therapies for opioid addictions. At the same time, flumazenil (Anexate, Canexat, Mazican, etc.) is available for benzodiazepine overdoses. The worsening of the opioid crisis during the 21st century led to a reexamining of U.S. sentencing guidelines during the Obama administration:

> On April 10, 2014, the United States Sentencing Commission voted unanimously to reduce the applicable sentencing guideline range for most federal drug trafficking offenses. The Amendment, often referred to as the "Drug Minus Two Amendment," reduced by two levels the base offense levels assigned by the Drug Quantity Table for each drug quantity, across all drug types. The Amendment became effective November 1, 2014.
>
> Separately, on July 18, 2014, the Commission unanimously voted to give retroactive effect to the Drug Minus Two Amendment, thereby allowing eligible offenders serving a previously imposed term of imprisonment to file a motion under 18 U.S.C. 3582 (c)(2) for a sentence reduction. The Commission's action allowed courts to begin considering such motions on November 1, 2014, but delayed the effective date of any sentence reduction orders until a year later, November 1, 2015. Since then (2020), courts have granted 30,852 retroactivity motions, resulting in an estimated average sentence reduction of 17.2 percent, from 146 to 121 months.[15]

The opioid crisis of the 21st century and the search for effective drug treatment alternatives led to a move toward weakening consent agreements between researchers and human subjects. The 21st Century Cures Act, passed by the 114th U.S. Congress in December 2016, essentially waived the consent requirement in certain studies where little harm was expected including those experiments involving veterans or active-duty personnel. The DOD research guidelines operate under the U.S. Code for the Armed Forces (10 USC 980) since 1956 now allows a waiver of advanced informed consent on the use of human subjects if the research shows minimal risks to the subjects and if the research project advances the development of a medical product necessary to the military. These conditions differ from those in effect at the time of the Tuskegee and similar studies in that research must now be carried out under all laws and regulations specified by the FDA.[16]

Under Section 3024 of the 21st Century Cures Act, researchers are allowed to waive informed consent requirements when their research purports to offers no or minimal risk coupled with adequate safeguards to the safety and welfare of human subjects. The Act provided 6.3 billion funding for clinical trials through the National Institutes of Health (NIH). The dire need for new drugs to counter both the opioid and COVID-19 crises also allows for companies to bypass randomized controlled trials for promising drugs and/or medical devices. Ironically, this measure was strongly supported by and lobbied for by the large pharmaceutical firms—the same firms alleged to have failed to adequately report the deadly side effects of opioid pain medications.[17]

The rush toward finding opioid antagonists and nonaddictive pain medicines in order to stem the tide of the opioid crisis provided the impetus for passage of the 21st Century Cures Act. The Act also assisted in the search for an effective treatment and/or immunization for the worldwide COVID-19 pandemic. Nonetheless, the blatant failure of the major drug companies to disclose the dangerous side effects of their popular and profitable pain medicines, notably Hydrocodone, OxyContin, and Fentanyl, has resulted in a number of law suits. And while there is evidence that these dangerous side effects were deliberately obscured from clinical trials, most of these cases remain within the civil, and not criminal, jurisdictions. Indeed, the three largest drug distributors, McKesson Corporation; Cardinal Health, Incorporated; and Amerisource Bergen Corporation, agreed in October 2019 to pay hundreds of millions of dollars in settlements for the unchecked distribution of tens of billions of opioid pills between 2006 and 2012 that fueled the massive opioid crisis in the United States. Also being sued in civil litigations is Purdue Pharm and the Sackler Family, the maker of OxyContin: "A recent lawsuit representing over 500 cities, counties and tribes accuse Purdue and eight members of the family, who deny wrongdoing, of misleading the public about the drug and profiting from the crisis ..."[18] While none of the Big Pharm leaders have been charged under the RICO laws like their illicit drug traffickers, the Sackler family has suffered considerable shame with their name, once prominently displayed at galleries, museums, and colleges and universities, now being removed.[19]

Notes

1 *Kefauver-Harris Act*. Public Law 87-781; 76 Stat. 780: 788–789 (October 10, 1962).
2 *Ibid.*
3 See Peltzma, S. 1973. An Evaluation of Consumer Protection Legislation: The 1962 Drug Amendments. *The Journal of Political Economy*, Vol. 81 (5) (September–October), p. 1051; Abood, R.R., & Brushwood, D.B. 1994. *Pharmacy Practice and the Law.* Gaithersburg, MD: Aspen Publishers, Inc.
4 See Milgram, S. 1974. *Obedience to Authority.* New York, NY: Harper & Row; Haney, C., Banks, W.C., & Zimbardo, P.G. 1973. A Study of Prisoners and Guards in a Simulated Prison. *Naval Research Review*, Vol. 30, pp. 4–17; Greenfield, R. 2006. *Timothy Leary: A Biography.* Boston, MA: Houghton-Mifflin Harcourt.
5 Welsome, E. 1999. *The Plutonium Files: America's Secret Medical Experiments in the Cold War.* New York, NY: The Dial Press/Random House.
6 Wiegand, T.J. 2007. Captive subjects: Pharmaceutical Testing and Prisoners, *Journal of Medical Toxicology*, Vol. 3 (1) (April), pp. 37–39.
7 Charles, A., & Draper, H. 2012. "Equivalence of Care" in Prison Medicine: Is Equivalence of Process the Right Measure of Equity. *Journal of Medical Ethics*, Vol. 38 (4) (April), pp. 215–218.
8 See www.VA.gov; *The Department of Veterans Act of 1988* (Public Law 100-527).
9 Rivers, P.C. 1994. *Alcohol and Human Behavior: Theory, Research, and Practice.* Englewood Cliffs, NJ: Prentice-Hall.
10 Rorabaugh, W.J. 1979. *The Alcohol Republic: An American Tradition.* New York, NY: Oxford University Press.
11 *Ibid.*, p. 14.
12 See *Chinese Exclusion Act of 1882*. U.S. Statutes at Large, 22 Stat. 58 (May 5); *Harrison Narcotics Tax Act of 1914*. Public Law 63-223. Stat. 38-785 (December 17).
13 Williams, J.C. 1990. *The Protectors: Anslinger and the Federal Bureau of Narcotics—1930–1962.* Newark, DE: University of Delaware Press; Sloan, L. 1979. *History of Marijuana in America.* Indianapolis, IN: Bobbs-Merrill; Burrough, B. 2004. *Public Enemies: America's Greatest Crime Wave and the Birth of the FBI: 1933–34.* New York, NY: Penguin Books; Gentry, G. 1991. *J. Edgar Hoover: The Man and the Secrets.* New York, NY: W.W. Norton & Company.
14 See *Anti-Drug Abuse Act of 1988*. Public Law 100-690. 102 Stat. 4181 (November 18).
15 Breyer, C.R., Reeves, D.C., Cushwa, P.K., & Wong, C.D. 2020. *Retroactivity & Recidivism: The Drugs Minus Two Amendment.* Washington, DC: U.S. Sentencing Commission (July).
16 See 10 U.S. Code 980, *Limitation on Use of Humans as Experimental Subjects.* Cornell Law School, Legal information Institute. Law.
17 See *21st Century Cures Act*. Public Law 114-255 (December 13, 2016).
18 Haynes, S. 2019. Sackler Family Philanthropy: Museums Cut Long Standing Ties. *Time* (April 8), p. 11.
19 *Ibid.*

5

DUTY TO WARN AND REPORT

The classic case relevant to the duty to protect the public, e.g., "duty to warn and report," was the 1974 *Tarasoff v. Regents of the University of California* and subsequently expanded to include child abuse and, more recently, police misconduct (duty to intervene) in the wake of the Black Lives Matter (BLM) movement.

The Duty to Warn: Exceptions to Client's Right to Confidentiality

Tarasoff v. Regents of the University of California. The Tarasoff case involves both the clinical and legal realms as well as university settings. It challenged the long-held concept of client privileges, a foundation stone of both the medical/clinical and legal disciplines. This case like many discussed in this work involves the discipline of psychology, most notably the failure of UC Berkeley's psychologist Dr. Lawrence (Larry) Moore, a clinician at the university's Cowell Memorial Hospital. Both the victim, Tatiana Tarasoff, and the offender, Prosenjit Poddar, were students at UC Berkeley in 1968 where Poddar held a strong romantic interest in Tarasoff that was not reciprocated. This unrequited relationship resulted in emotional stress bringing Poddar to the attention of Dr. Moore at the university's Cowell Clinic in 1969.

Within this clinical milieu, Poddar disclosed homicidal ideations toward Tarasoff at which time Dr. Moore provided a possible diagnosis of paranoid schizophrenia. Accordingly, he knew that the seriousness of this disorder warranted breeching client/therapist confidentiality due to its potential for harm to Tarasoff or Poddar's suicide. Dr. Moore subsequently notified the campus police suggesting Poddar be hospitalized. Campus police interviewed Poddar and released him while, Dr. Harvey Powelson, Dr. Moore's immediate supervisor as well as the director of Psychiatry at Cowell Memorial Hospital, ordered Moore's notes on Poddar be destroyed. No one from the Moore Clinic or law enforcement warned Tatiana Tarasoff or her parents of the threats against her. Poddar continued to stalk her and killed her on October 27, 1969.[1]

Tatiana's parents sued the Regents of the University of California in the state court where the lower court dismissed the case siding with the defendants who claimed that their responsibility was to maintain the confidentiality of their client, Prosenjit Poddar. The Tarasoff family appealed

DOI: 10.4324/9781003224426-5

the lower court decision to the California Supreme Court which sided with the plaintiffs in its 1974 decision. The California ruling again reaffirmed this ruling in 1976 setting the stage for major changes within professional ethics as well as establishing a precedent for subsequent similar civil cases. Melton discussed the clinical/legal implications of the Tarasoff decision in the area of forensic psychology in his book, *Psychological Evaluations for the Courts*:

> Although most jurisdictions now recognize a *Tarasoff*-type duty, the vast majority that do limit it to situations in which, to use the words of the California statute enacted after *Tatasoff*, "the patient has communicated to the psychotherapist a serious threat of physical violence against a reasonably identifiable victim or victims." Moreover, application of the duty to therapists does not necessarily mean it also applies to evaluators, even in those situations where the attorney-client privilege would permit disclosure. A person does not normally have a legal obligation to help another unless he or she stands in a "special relationship" to that person ... There is evidence to suggest that *Tarasoff* has inhibited the therapeutic process and that applying its rule to either the therapeutic or evaluative context does more harm than good. On the other hand, the American Psychiatric Association has indicated it may be proper to hold a psychiatrist liable for "flagrant negligent" failures to protect others from harm, and ethical rules mandate a duty to protect the public.[2]

Again there is not unanimous agreement on what psychologists and other clinician should do in situations such as Tarasoff. A leading psychologist at the time, Max Siegel (1983 American Psychological Association [APA] President), led the group that saw client/therapist confidentiality as a paramount ethical standard that should not be breeched under any circumstances. Ironically, during Siegel's reign as APA President, another California case, *Jablonski by Pahls v. United States*, was being decided by the 9th U.S. Circuit of Appeals. This was a federal case given that it involved a doctor at the Loma Linda Veterans Administration Hospital. Philip Carl Jablonski, a U.S. Army Vietnam veteran (1966–1968), was evaluated at the Veteran Affairs (VA) facility following a serious domestic attack on his then live-in girlfriend, the mother of his child. The VA assessment did not go beyond the basic Tarasoff guidelines of warning the potential victim. Jablonski, who already had a record of violent sexual assaults, subsequently killed Melinda Kimball. Sentenced to 12 years for Kimball's death, he was paroled early and went on to kill more intimate partners and significant others. In all, Jablonski is credited with the murder of five women between 1978 and 1991. He received the death sentence in 1994 for the murder of Fathyma Vann in 1991. He died at San Quentin Prison on December 27, 2019, at age 73.

This case intersects with the quality of care at federal VA facilities which were dealing with an onslaught of post-traumatic stress disorder (PTSD) cases afflicting Vietnam veterans. Although only recently recognized as a serious form of trauma, PTSD was recognized as a viable mental disorder in 1980 under the new *Diagnostic and Statistical Manual for Mental Disorders* (*DSM-III*). Even then, the VA, during the Reagan administration, was not encouraged to rigorously pursue mental health claims from Vietnam veterans. Thus, the clinician at the Loma Linda VA Hospital did what was the expected status quo regarding its evaluation and assessment of Philip Carl Jablonski. However, the 9th U.S. Circuit Court of Appeals found that the duty to warn went beyond the Tarasoff decision and that in order to predict "dangerousness," mental health evaluations needed to include prior records and, when dangerousness is determined, to take action to protect potential victims including having the client placed under involuntary emergency hospital care until definitive clinical and legal actions can be better ascertained.[3]

Seven years following Tatiana Tarasoff's death, another co-ed death, Jeanne Clery, led to an expansion of the Tarasoff and Jablonski duty to warn decisions. Jeanne Clery, a 19-year-old co-ed at Lehigh University in Bethlehem Pennsylvania, was raped and murdered in her residence hall by a fellow student, Joseph, in 1986. Her parents, like that of Tatiana Tarasoff, litigation leveled against the university led to passage of the 1990 *Security Policy and Campus Crime Statistics Act, aka—the "Clery Act."* The Clery Act initiated a review of other campuses where violent crimes were basically hidden from law enforcement and the public in order to protect the university or college image. The Clery Act cited serious violations at a number of schools, including Penn State, Eastern Michigan, Virginia Tech, and the University of Montana. The Clery Act required that all colleges and universities in the United States that participate in federal financial aid programs (the vast majority of institutions of higher education) maintain a record of campus crimes and disclose this information each October 1 in a "Annual Campus Security Report."[4]

It is important to note sociocultural factors surrounding the Tarasoff and Clery "duty to warn" cases as they pertain to academic institutions. Both cases involved White co-eds and minority offenders of color—Poddar was of India's lower caste, while Henry was African-American. Serious crimes on American campuses were not new but apparently it took an interracial event to mount enough interest to lead to major changes in how these matters were handled. Racial tensions were high from the 1960s through the 1980s with the Civil Rights and Anti-War Movements and later with school desegregation. The Tarasoff case occurred in the California Bay Area, the epicenter for both the "Hippies" and the "Black Panthers," while the Clery case happened on Frank Rizzo's racist turf where the widespread fears of White women being raped and murdered by Black strangers was perpetrated through the works of Marvin Wolfgang at the University of Pennsylvania. What the public was not aware of is that neither of these cases involved an "outsider" coming onto the campus for the purpose of rape and murder. Also lacking at that time was an understanding of sociocultural factors such as social class, differential socialization, gender relations and expectations, etc. In Poddar's case, his second-degree murder conviction was over, and he was deported back to India where he apparently married and lived his life without further incidents. It is easy to understand Dr. Moore's preliminary diagnosis of paranoid schizophrenia given that therapists were not adequately alerted to cultural variants in clinical diagnoses until the emergence of the *DSM-III* in 1980. With the anti-Black sentiments prevalent at the time of his original trial, the death sentence issued to Joseph M. Henry in the Clery case was challenged on appeal in 2002 at which time Henry accepted a life sentence in lieu of going through another trial where he could again receive the death sentence.[5] Yet another critical sociocultural factor of the time was the HIV-AIDS crisis notably among gay males. The issue here was does the duty to warn involving the clients right to privacy and confidentiality supersede the duty to warn potential victims? This medical/legal quandary led to passage of the "Standards for Privacy of Identifiable Health Information" (Privacy Rule) element of the Health Insurance Portability and Accountability Act of 1996.[6]

Duty to Report

The *Tarasoff* and *Clery* cases illustrated abuses within institutions of higher learning and its college-age cohort. Child abuse of minors was another important arena for professionals (teachers, doctors/clinicians, clergy, etc.) to not only warn but to report any suspected abuse among those minors they interacted within their official capacity. The "Child Abuse Prevention and Treatment Act" (CAPTA) was initiated in the 1970s in the same era of the Tarasoff case. CAPTA became effective January 31, 1974, as Public Law 93-247:

AN ACT: To provide financial assistance for a demonstration program for the prevention, identification, and treatment of child abuse and neglect, to establish a National Center on Child Abuse and Neglect, and for other purposes.

SEC. 3. For the purpose of this Act the term "child abuse and neglect" means the physical or mental injury, sexual abuse, negligent treatment, or maltreatment of a child under the age of eighteen by a person who is responsible for the child's welfare under circumstances which indicate that the child's health or welfare is prescribed by the Secretary (Secretary of Health, Education, and Welfare; now Secretary of Health and Human Services).

SEC. 4 (2). In order for a State to qualify for assistance under this subsection, such State shall-

(A) have in effect a State child abuse and neglect law which shall include provisions for immunity for persons reporting instances of child abuse and neglect from prosecution, under any State or local law, arising out of such reporting;
(B) provide for the reporting of known and suspected instances of child abuse and neglect;
(C) provide that upon receipt of a report of known or suspected instances of child abuse or neglect an investigation shall be initiated promptly to substantiate the accuracy of the report, and, upon finding of abuse or neglect, immediate steps shall be taken to protect the health and welfare of the abused or neglected child, as well as that of any other child under the same care who may be in danger of abuse or neglect;
(D) demonstrate that there are in effect throughout the State, in connection with the enforcement of child abuse and neglect laws and with the reporting of suspected instances of child abuse and neglect, such administrative procedures, such personnel trained in child abuse and neglect prevention and treatment, such training procedures, such institutional and other facilities (public and private), and such related multidisciplinary programs and services as may be necessary or appropriate to assure that the State will deal effectively with child abuse and neglect cases in the State;
(E) provide for methods to preserve the confidentiality of all records in order to protect the rights of the child, his parents or guardians;
(F) provide for the cooperation of law enforcement officials, courts of competent jurisdictions, and appropriate State agencies providing human services;
(G) provide that in every case involving an abused or neglected child which results in a judicial proceeding a guardian ad litem shall be appointed to represent the child in such proceedings.[7]

Adaptations to the original 1974 CAPTA were instituted in 1988 (Public Law 100-247) relevant to the establishment of a National Center on Child Abuse with the new title of "Child Abuse Prevention, Adoption and Family Services Act of 1988." The most recent CAPTA adaptation was incorporated in the Comprehensive Addiction and Recovery Act of 2016.[8] These additions aside, the basic CAPTA rules initiated in 1974 remain in effect, that is, that every U.S. State and Territory needs to have laws regulating the reporting of suspected child abuse and neglect cases. The United States being a federal-form of government, major changes such as this requires either a Constitutional Amendment or a monetary incentive in order to entice States and Territories to comply. Here it was the monetary incentive that got the program off the ground. That said, there is no federal template that applies to all the States and Territories, other than the general reporting guidelines and some form of immunity for those reporting suspected incidents of child abuse or neglect. A common response is for States to pass reporting laws whereby a failure to do so could result in a misdemeanor offense. In New Mexico, I trained teachers, social workers, psychologists/mental health counselors, and police academy personnel on the State's reporting laws and the consequences for noncompliance (misdemeanor offense). The New Mexico statute required that suspected abuse or neglect be reported within 48 hours to either the police or to a state social welfare agency. Those reporting suspected child abuse or neglect could do so anonymously. Given the high caseload for state social workers, I recommended that law enforcement should be contacted first. The rationale being that police departments were compelled to notify the welfare agency within the 48-hour time frame for initiating action. This process facilitated the reporting time frame even though there likely would be a delay in action from the welfare office.[9]

Federal Omission—Indian Country

While the federal child abuse and neglect initiative was being pushed upon the States and Territories, it did not apply to federal jurisdictions, most notably Indian Country. This would only come about following the 1989 Special Committee on Investigations of the 101st Congress in a report entitled *A New Federalism for American Indians*. What was unique is that while existing State statutes are designed to report suspected incidents of domestic violence, that is often shrouded in the privacy of home settings, the federal statute unfolded yet another significant dimension of child abuse and neglect—that perpetrated by professionals trusted with the care and welfare of children and youth. Clearly, a federal child abuse and neglect reporting mandate was paramount given the dire, often grossly underfunded, conditions existing on federally supervised tribes comprising the vast semi-autonomous tracks across America known collectively as "Indian Country." Indian Country was, and continues to be, a cauldron of misery, poverty, unemployment, poor health care, and domestic violence. It took abuses by federally hired teachers and negligence at the hands of Bureau of Indian Affairs (BIA) officials to illustrate the nature and extent of this problem which is provided in the Report's Executive Summary:

> The Committee found that the BIA (Bureau of Indian Affairs) also permitted a pattern of child abuse by its teachers to fester throughout BIA schools nationwide. For almost 15 years, while child reporting standards were being adopted by all 50 states, the Bureau failed to issue any reporting guidelines for its own teachers. Incredibly, the BIA did not even require even a minimum background check into potential school employees. As a result, the BIA employed teachers who actually admitted past child molestation, including at least one Arizona teacher who explicitly listed a prior criminal offense for child abuse on his employment form.
>
> At a Cherokee Reservation (Quall Boundary—Eastern Band of Cherokee Indians) elementary school in North Carolina, the BIA employed Paul Price, another confessed child molester—even after his previous principal, who had fired him for molesting seventh grade boys, warned BIA officials that Price was an admitted pedophile. Shocked to learn several years later from teachers at the Cherokee school that Price continued to teach despite the warning, Price's former principal told several Cherokee teachers of Price's pedophilia and notified the highest BIA official in Cherokee. Instead of dismissing Price or conducting an inquiry, BIA administrators lectured an assembly of Cherokee teachers on the unforeseen consequences of slander.
>
> The Committee found that during his 14 years at Cherokee, Price molested at least 25 students while the BIA continued to ignore repeated allegations—including an eyewitness account by a teacher's aide. Even after Price was finally caught and the negligence of BIA supervisors came to light, not a single official was ever disciplined for tolerating the abuse

> of countless students for 14 years. Indeed, the negligent Cherokee principal who received the eyewitness report was actually promoted to the BIA Central Office in Washington—the same office which, despite the Price case, failed for years to institute background checks for potential teachers or reporting requirements for instances of suspected abuse. Another BIA Cherokee school official was promoted to the Hopi Reservation in Arizona without any inquiry into his handling of the Price fiasco.
>
> Meanwhile at Hopi (Pueblo), a distraught mother reported to the local BIA principal a possible instance of child sexual abuse by the remedial reading teacher, John Boone. Even though five years earlier the principal had received police records of alleged child sexual abuse by Boone, the principal failed to investigate the mother's report or contact law enforcement authorities. He simply notified his superior, who also took no action. A year later, the same mother eventually reported the teacher to the FBI (Federal Bureau of Investigation), which found that he had abused 142 Hopi children, most during the years of BIA's neglect. Again, no discipline or censure of school officials followed: the BIA simply provided the abused children with one counsellor who compounded their distress by intimately interviewing them for a book he wished to write on the case.
>
> Sadly, these wrongs were not isolated incidents. While in the past year the Bureau has finally promulgated some internal child abuse reporting guidelines, it has taken the Special Committee's public hearing for the BIA to fully acknowledge its failures.[10]

In reaction to the Select Committee's findings, the U.S. Congress passed *The Indian Child Abuse Prevention and Treatment Act* in 1990. The Bill established mandatory reporting procedures for certain professionals working in Indian Country by amending Title 18 of the U.S. Code, providing criminal penalties for failure to report cases of child abuse or neglect holding Indian Country to the same rules regulating child protection as that in State jurisdictions:

> The Select Committee on Indian Affairs and the Special Committee on Investigations have held numerous hearings which focused on the growing problem of child abuse and neglect in Indian country ... The hearings of the Special Committee on Investigations focused primarily on three reservations, Navajo, Hopi, and Cherokee which have suffered cases of child sexual abuse where large number of children were abused over a period of years ...
>
> Section 1 of the Bill establishes mandatory reporting procedures for certain professionals working in Indian country by amending Title 18 of the United States Code and providing criminal penalties for failure to report cases of child abuse or neglect. The Committee is very concerned that the reluctance of professionals working in Indian country to report instances of child sexual abuse must be corrected. The Committee has heard much testimony from tribal witnesses regarding their frustrations with the lack of timely prosecution of cases of child sexual abuse in Indian country. In many cases, Indian tribes have been unable to proceed with prosecutions in tribal court in cases of child sexual abuse where the United States Attorneys have declined prosecutions, or because of breakdowns in communications with the United States Attorney in United States District Courts ...
>
> Section 4(a)(1) sets out the reporting procedures for cases of child abuse and neglect in Indian country. This section would amend Title 18 of the United States Code to include a section 1169, which would establish mandatory reporting requirements.
>
> Under subsection(a) of 1169, if a person who is a physician, teacher, administrative officer of any public or private school, social worker, psychiatrist, child counsellor, mental health

> professional, law enforcement officer, or other identified person, knows or has reasonable suspicion that a child was abused or neglected in Indian country and fails to immediately report such abuse or neglect to a local child protective services agency or local law enforcement agency, that person shall be subject to a fine of up to $5,000 or imprisonment of not more than six months, or both.
>
> Subsection (b) of 1169 provides that any person who supervises or has authority over a person described in subsection (a) and inhibits or prevents that person from reporting a case of abuse or neglect shall be subject to a fine of up to $5,000 or imprisonments of not more than six months, or both.
>
> Subsection (d)(2) of 1169 provides that any local enforcement agency shall immediately notify the local child protective services agency and shall submit copies of the written reports required under section (c) to said agency. Section 4(b)(2) provides that any local child protective services agency shall immediately notify the local law enforcement agency and shall submit copies of the written reports required under subsection (c) to said agency. This section also provides that where the Federal Bureau of Investigation (FBI) has jurisdiction, the Bureau shall receive immediate notice of the child abuse.[11]

The Eastern Band of Cherokee Indians (Qualla Band) passed an ordinance that augmented the federal Indian Child Abuse Prevention and Treatment Act by banishing enrolled tribal members from their Indian trust lands who are convicted of a sexual offense against a minor on the reservation. Subsequent action could lead to being officially removed from the tribal rolls.[12]

Child abuse and neglect among American Indians under government protection was not limited to the United States. Indeed, Canada often mimicked American Indian policies and practices with equally devastating effects. Canada's abuse of its indigenous peoples extended back to the late 1800s when the government contracted with churches to run the compulsory Indian Residential Boarding Schools. Here, the churches (Roman Catholic, Presbyterian, United Church of Canada, and the Anglican Church of Canada) were mandated to destroy any remnants of aboriginal culture through a harsh process of pseudo assimilation—pseudo in that full membership into Canadian society was not an intent or option for First Nations, Inuit, or Mete until 1982. Physical, mental, and sexual abuse abounded within this environment which existed until the mid-1970s involving some 150,000 Indian children and youth. Other elements of child abuse and neglect, including sexual abuse, existed in other venues including incidents within parishes and congregations as well as in orphanages and schools operated by the Christian Brothers in British Columbia and Newfoundland. Numerous law suits have been since filed by those tribal members wronged during this era of blatant abuse. These legal actions have impacted financially on these religious orders much like the current impact upon the Roman Catholic Church worldwide.[13]

Child abuse and neglect issues have dominated the news over the past 30 years with more horrid tales of sexual abuse within established institutions including schools, religious groups, athletic organizations, and even the Boy Scouts of America. Perhaps the most visible cases involve the Roman Catholic Church brought forth by an expose by the *Boston Globe*, which exposed child sexual abuse by parish priests in Massachusetts. The January 2002 Pulitzer Prize-winning *Boston Globe* article, "Church allowed abuse of priest for years: Aware of Geoghan record, archdiocese still shuttled him from parish," ignited a firestorm of rage in the United State initially setting off a chain of investigations worldwide—Canada, Ireland, the United Kingdom, Mexico, Belgium, France, Germany, and Australia; and later in Africa and South and Central America with Father John J. Geoghan as the personification of pedophilia within the church.[14] The United States Conference of Catholic Bishops (USCCB) initiated a study under the direction of the John Jay

College of Criminal Justice to ascertain the prevalence of the problem in the United States for the period 1950 until 2002. The results indicated over 10,000 minor victims with the vast majority (80%) being male. More than 4,000 priests were implicated in the study comprising about 4% of the over 100,000 priests in active ministry during this time frame. Of this cohort, 149 priests accounted for more than 25% of all identified victims.[15] The alarm directed toward the Roman Catholic Church was the issue of the above average percentage of suspected homosexual priests. The John Jay College report, as well as other studies, indicates that up to a third of Catholic priests are admittedly homosexuals. While this does not imply that they actively seek out sexual liaisons with other gay men or, for those that do, that their preference are children and youth. Adding to the homosexual priest stigma is the tendency to label them as potential pedophiles.[16]

It became evident that this was not merely a problem with Roman Catholic clergy, the prevalence of child and adolescent sexual abuse afflicted many other denominations as the Canadian study reveals. The issue of abuse by professionals entrusted with the protection of children and youth is similar to that which was exposed within the Indian schools in both the United States and Canada. The major difference was that the U.S. Indian Commission report was not widely disseminated and therefore gained little public attention. The Catholic clergy abuse, on the other hand, was widely distributed. A common theme in both instances is the seemingly premeditated breech of ethics by those professionals who abuse dependent children and youth dependent upon their care and protection. A yet-to-be-resolved problem within society is the portrayal of perpetrators of child abuse, notably sexual abuse, as pedophiles—a label that carries the worst stigma of any abuse short of murder.

Paraphilias differ markedly from people who find those dependent upon their care as convenient fodder for their sexual outlet. Paraphilias represent a rare but serious form of mental illness, one of impulse-control dysregulation: an endogenous process involving the greater limbic system, notably the "hypothalamic-pituitary-adrenal-gonad axis" in males. Like other impulse-control disorders (the *manias*), the primary objective of this autonomic process is impersonal sexual gratification. The most dangerous type of paraphilia is males who seem helpless in overriding these impulsive sexual urges with pedophiliacs targeting pre-pubic children. Contrary to popular belief, increased testosterone levels are not the primary factor in these recurring, intense, sexually arousing fantasies. On the contrary, marked levels of testosterone are more likely to be associated with irritability and aggression rather than with sexual desires. Reduction in serum testosterone has a similar effect on both men and women—a reduction in their libido. It is the luteinizing hormone (LH) that is closely associated with sexual fantasies in males as it is with the undesired effects of premenstrual syndrome (PMS) with females. In males, LH stimulates the sexual fantasies which become compulsive, and often dangerous, among paraphiliacs: a process that has a powerful control over a person's affect often overriding frontal-lobe cognitive capacities resulting in intense sexually arousing fantasies and sexual urges that tend to depersonalize or objectify the victim. Other paraphilias that have a potential for dangerousness include sexual masochism and sexual sadism.[17]

While paraphilia presents as a pervasive impulse-control disorder that is difficult to treat or self-regulate, most sexual offenses fall within the area of a sex-stress situation which is often driven by environmental and interpersonal variables. Sexual behavior precipitated by social/environmental/familial stressors falls under the general classification of "sex-stress situations." These are impulsive sexual acts involving stimuli that trigger intense levels of excitability—anger, revenge, paranoid ideations, a sense of entitlement, and the like. These acts generally target specific persons and can be associated with diminished cognitive capacity often associated with substance use or abuse. These acts can be dangerous resulting in serious sexual abuse and even death. Sex-stress situations account for forcible rape and similar offenses while what historically was known as statutory rape is sexual behavior prohibited by law involving consenting partners where one is not of the legal age to offer consent. An important distinction is that paraphilia is a serious mental health issue that has indigenous roots thus transcending mere cognitive therapeutic approaches. On the other hand, variants of sex-stress situations, in most cases, involve transitory impulses that can be addressed clinically through cognitive behavioral therapy. The clinical/legal dilemma is compounded by the trend in the United States to legislate "childhood." The standard biological definition of life stages is divided into pre-public children and adolescence and the various stages of adulthood. Someone sexually fixated on pre-pubic infants and children is clinically termed to be a pedophile. Once puberty has been reached and boys and girls start to manifest physical attributes that clearly identify their sexual development, they should no longer be clinically labeled as "children" but rather as pre-teens, teens, youth, or adolescents. The biological/legal dilemma stems from the fact that official status is legislated by individual states and does not necessarily follow biological, medical, or clinical criteria.[18]

The tendency in the United States is to view all sex offenders as being cut from the same bolt of cloth, crafting laws that do not discern between social problems and clinical pathologies. Legislating sexual status in itself is not consistent within States where in some jurisdictions the age for charging someone as an adult and therefore being tried in criminal court is 13 while at the same time labeling sexual abuse victims under age 18 as "children" allowing for more serious charges to be brought against the alleged offender. This confusion has led to a serious backlash in the United States toward sex offenders often with a vigilante mentality placing convicted sex offenders under greater scrutiny and harassment that even murders. Part of the problem is that state and federal laws often do not distinguish between consensual sex among teens/young adults and dangerous sexual offenders. In these jurisdictions, there is a clear lack of science-based distinctions made between classifications of paraphilias, notably pedophilia. "Megan's Law" illustrated this divide. Megan's Law resulted as a national outcry over the rape and murder of seven-year-old Megan Kanka in New Jersey in 1994. Megan's Law resulted in public disclosure laws requiring the whereabouts of convicted sex offenders leading to the creation of a national registration center with failure to register constituting a felony-level offense. At the federal level, the Center for Sex Offender Management was established in 1997 within the U.S. Department of Justice (DOJ). Abuse by clergy, notably Roman Catholics, has also hastened the cry for more severe retribution for those labeled as dangerous sexual offenders. This outcry has led to the call for post-sentencing incarceration termed, "sexual predator laws," often resulting in de facto life sentences.

Equally compelling are compulsory reporting laws that effectively render labeled offenders homeless once released from serving their sex abuse sentence. These severe sanctions are dictated under the U.S. DOJ guidelines known as the *Sex-Offender Registration and Notification Act* (SORNA) that took effect in July 2009. All state jurisdictions are required to use the SORNA tiering system in classifying sex offenders whereby the minimum registration period for tier I offenders is 15 years; tier II offenders, 25 years; and lifetime registration for tier III offenders. Under this mandate, offenders must notify the jurisdiction of any change of name, residence, employment, or student status, in person, no later than three business days following any of these changes in their status. Failure to do so constitutes a felony offense in most jurisdictions.[19]

Additionally, many states have enacted civil commitment laws whereby a panel of "professionals" determine if a convicted sex offender can be kept institutionalized in forensic settings beyond the fulfillment of their criminal sentence. Other jurisdictions have forced released sex offenders to live rough away from any public housing, schools, parks, libraries, etc. Efforts have even been made in some states to death qualify sex offenders, attempting to expand the death sentence beyond that of special categories of homicide. In comparison, Canada which shares some of the worse abuse of compulsory Indian boarding schools with the United States has a model that differs markedly from that of America. Most importantly, the general public does not have access to the sex-offender registry like that in the United States. Moreover, sex offenses are prosecuted at the federal level under the authority of the North America Act of 1867 where the government is responsible for enacting criminal law and procedures with the provinces having the responsibility of administrating said laws. Hence, Canada promulgated laws dealing with *criminal sexual psychopaths* in 1948 with indeterminate sentences of between 4- and 14-year incarceration. In 1997, the long-term offender (LTO) section was applied to sex offenders who were deemed to be at risk of reoffending allowing for community supervision for up to 10 years. Canada instituted its *Sex Offender Information Registration Act* (SOIRA) ahead of the United States. Their registry differs markedly from the United States' SORNA in that the Canadian registry is accessible only to Canadian law enforcement personnel and is administered by the Royal Canadian Mounted Police (RCMP, aka *Mounties*). The SOIRA criteria correspond with the sex offender's sentence with a 10-year registration for sentences of 2–5 years; 20 years for sentences of 10–14 years; and a lifetime registration requirement for longer sentences and/or repeat offenders. Life time registrants can apply for a judicial review at 5-year intervals.[20]

The cases of child abuse and neglect, including sexual abuse and homicide, resulted in the emergence of laws relevant to the duty to warn and the duty to report such abuse both in the United States and Canada. This action took place in the 1970s with the Tarasoff case and continued to the present as continued focus is placed on clergy abuse and abuse within the Boys Scouts. Added dimensions of duty to report and warn are covered later in the book in cases resulting from the *Me Too* and the *BLM* movements of the early 21st century.

Notes

1 *Tarasoff v. Regents, University of California*, 551 P.2d 334 (Cal. 1976).
2 Melton, G.B., Petrila, J., Plytghress, N.C., & Slobogin, C. 1997. The Duty to Protect the Public (Tarasoff), *Psychological Evaluations for the Courts: A Handbook for Mental Health Professionals and Lawyers* (2nd ed.). New York, NY: The Guilford Press, pp. 76–77.
3 See *Jablonski by Pahls v. United States,* 712 F.2d 391 (9th Cir. 1983); Mills, M.J., Sullivan, G., & Eth, S. 1987. Protecting third parties: a decade after Tarasoff. *American Journal of Psychiatry,* Vol. 144 (1), pp. 68–74.
4 See *Security Policy and Campus Crime Statistics Act of 1990.* Public Law 101-542, U.S. Code of Federal Regulations, 34 C.F.R. 668.46 20 USC 1092.
5 Blum, D. 1986. *Bad Karma: A True Story of Obsession and Murder.* New York, NY: Atheneum; French, L.A. 2018. *The History of Policing America: From Militias and Military to the Law Enforcement of Today.* Lanham, MD: Rowman & Littlefield.
6 See *Health Insurance Portability and Accountability Act of 1996.* "Standards for Privacy of Identifiable Health Information" (Privacy Rule) finalized March 2002. Public Law 104-191; 45 CFR Part 160 ^ 164.
7 *Child Abuse Prevention and Treatment Act.* Public Law 93-247; 42 USC 101; January 31, 1974 (S. 1191).
8 See *Comprehensive Addiction and Recovery Act of 2016* (CARA). Public Law 114-198 (July 22, 2016).
9 See *Mandatory Reporters of Child Abuse and Neglect.* 2019. Washington, DC: U.S. Department of Health and Human Services, Children's Bureau.
10 *Final Report and Legislative Recommendations: A Report of the Special Committee on Investigations of the Select Committee on Indian Affairs* (November, 1989). U.S. Senate, Part One—The Executive Summary: A New Federalism for American Indians, 101st Congress, 1st Session, 101–160, 9–10. Washington, DC: U.S. Government Printing Office.
11 *Indian Child Protection and Family Violence Prevention Act, Title IV* (November 28, 1990). Public Law 101-630. 25 USC 3210.

12 See Eastern Band of Cherokee Indians, Tribal Resolution #59 (December 5, 1991).
13 Kondro, W. (1998). Canada Apologies to Native People Who Suffered Abuse. *The Lancet*, Vol. 351 (#9097) (17 January), p. 194.
14 See "Church allowed abuse by priests for years: Aware of Geoghan record, archdiocese still shuttled him from parish to parish," *Boston Globe* (January 2, 2002). www.bostonglobe.com/news/special-report/2002/01/06.
15 Berry, J., & Renner, G. 2004. *Vows of Silence: The Abuse of Power in the Papacy of John Paul II.* New York, NY: Free Press.
16 Jenkins, P. 2001. *Pedophiles and Priests: Anatomy of a Contemporary Crisis.* New York, NY: Oxford University Press; Guimaraes, A.S. 1999. *The Catholic Church and Homosexuality.* Charlotte, NC: Tan Books and Publications.
17 French, L.A. 1995. Treating the Dangerous Sexual Offender. *Sexual Issues in Counseling & Therapy* (Lesson 6). Long Island, NY: The Hatherleigh Company; *The Diagnostic and Statistical Manual of Mental Disorders—Fifth Edition* (DSM-5). 2013. American Psychiatric Association.
18 See Petrunik, M., & Deutschmann, L. 2007. The Exclusion-Inclusion Spectrum in State and Community Responses to Sex Offenders in Anglo-American and European Jurisdictions. *International Journal of Offender Therapy and Comparative Criminology*, Vol. 20 (10), pp. 1–21.
19 See U.S. SORNA. 2009. *Sex-Offenders Registration and Notification Act.* www.justice.gov/oig/reports/plus/e0901/Final.pdf.
20 See Canada SOIRA. 2004. *Sex Offender Information Registration Act.* http://novascotia.ca/pps/publications/camanual/ProsecutionPolicies/SOIRApolicy04.pdf.

6
CRUEL AND UNUSUAL

The Prevalence of Systemic Racism

Institutional racism, the roots of the current pervasive malaise, "systemic racism," is embedded in major professions, not only in the United States but worldwide. The privilege of professional status, if unchecked by independent ethics ombudsmen, can, and often, result in discrimination against perceived threatening "others." While elements of institutional racism are discussed in Chapter 2 as it pertains to "due process" within America's judicial ideals, this section looks at politically sanctioned, clandestine international applications of cruel and unusual practices deliberately devised to skirt American and international judicial protocols for political ends.

Again, the profession of psychology and noted psychologists are prominent players in this process especially as it pertains to the post-9/11/2001 *War on Terrorism* and America's worldwide pursuit of demonizing and punishing those deemed responsible for this infamous attack on the United States. The main issue is the tacit approval of the use of torture despite its universal ban. Prominent psychologists in the past who set the stage for psychological testing (Edward L. Thorndike, Robert M. Yerkes, Lewis M. Terman, Abraham H. Maslow), including those whose research on psychological manipulation (Kenneth B. Clark, Philip G. Zimbardo), set the stage for their elevation to the APA Presidency. This status was also conferred on Martin E.P. Seligman (1998 APA President) whose work on *Learned Helplessness* provided the basis for the CIA's human torture program. Seligman's concept of learned helplessness added to Abraham Maslow's earlier work regarding the hierarchy of human needs, a paradigm that provided the basis for *brain washing* yet another component of human torture.[1]

Seligman's work on learned helplessness postulated that subjects after being subjected repeatedly to aversive stimuli start to lose their sense of control. His research used dogs in a laboratory situation and not human subjects avoiding the pitfalls of Milgram and Zimbardo. Seligman and colleagues inferred from the lab research that, in humans, a lack of self-efficacy can be a major contributing factor in reactive depression for some. These insights led to the development of cognitive behavioral therapies where focus is placed on the factors people attributed to their depression. Seligman's work adds to the earlier work by Hans Selye's general adaptation syndrome (GAS) developed in 1936 at McGill University in Montreal, Canada. Inferring from laboratory rats to

DOI: 10.4324/9781003224426-6

humans, Selye demonstrated how pervasive stressful environments can impact the immune system contributing to both mental and physical health problems. Constant trauma engages the autonomic nervous system so that it over engages the adrenal "fight or flight" response without adequate para-sympatric replenishment contributing to fatigue, burnout, depression, anxiety, post-traumatic stress, etc. These insights into human behavior aided other psychologists in devising torture protocols for the U.S. government following the 9/11/01 terrorist attacks.[2]

International Conventions Against Torture

Protocols against torture and inhuman and cruel treatment are linked to wars and similar conflicts and are generally described within acceptable articles of war and martial law. Interestingly, the U.S. Civil War (1861–1865) provided the foundation for subsequent international conventions outlining unacceptable treatments of both prisoners of war (POWs) and captured civilian populations. The idea of universal human rights emerged as slavery was ending within Western cultures. Prior to the ending slavery, the treatment of one's property was seen as falling outside civil and criminal jurisdictions. It took an expanded definition of "human" to establish an agreed upon set of standards defining acceptable versus unacceptable behaviors within and between societies.

The "Lieber Code" was devised by Franz Lieber, a law school professor, with the influence of U.S. General Henry Halleck who previously published on the rules regulating the intercourse of States in peace and war. The Lieber Code was adopted by U.S. President Abraham Lincoln as General Order #100 for the Union forces in the Civil War. The Lieber Code became effective as the "code-of-conduct" for Union forces effective April 24, 1863. In addition to eliminating "no quarter" massacres of captures and forbidding rape, and spelling out specific rules of conduct regarding the treatment of spies, prisoners-of-war, and deserters, it addressed the treatment of Blacks lending itself to Lincoln's Emancipation Proclamation also issued in April 1863. It departed markedly from the Confederate policy of treating Black Union soldiers as criminals and not as soldiers, subject to summary execution or re-enslavement upon capture. A unique element of the Lieber Code is that it prohibited discrimination on the basis of color among combatants. Most importantly, the Lieber Code established the foundation for international regulations on customs of war, including a prohibition of torture, beginning with The Hague Regulations of 1907 which basically elevated the Lieber Code to the level of international law.[3]

The impetus for International Humanitarian Law (IHL) followed the atrocities committed during the World War II (WWII) on all sides, resulting in Geneva Convention of 1949. Critical to the 1907, 1949 and subsequent Geneva Conventions dealing with IHL was the prohibition of torture. Torture is also prohibited under International Human Rights Law (IHRL). The International Committee of the Red Cross (ICRC) defines torture and other forms of ill-treatment under the IHL and IHRL as follows:

1. Any act by which severe pain or suffering, whether physical or mental, is inflicted on a person;
2. The act must be intentionally inflicted;
3. The act must be instrumental for such purposes as:
   (a) obtaining from the individual or a third person information or a confession, or
   (b) punishing him/her for an act he/she or a third person has committed or is suspected of having committed, or
   (c) intimidating him/her or a third person, or
   (d) coercing him/her or a third person, or
   (e) for any reason based on discrimination of any kind.[4]

Accordingly, the ICRC defines "inhuman and cruel treatment" as the infliction of severe physical or mental pain or suffering, which goes beyond mere degradation or humiliation. Unlike torture, there is no requirement that inhuman and cruel treatment be inflicted for a specific purpose. A distinction between the IHL and the IHRL is that the former applies to all parties to an armed conflict, while the latter applies specifically to States. Additionally, the 1998 Rome Statute of the International Criminal Court (ICC) classified torture and other inhuman treatment (crimes against humanity) to be *war crimes* in both international and non-international armed conflicts. The United Nations (UN) Committee Against Torture (CAT) acts as an independent body with the mandate of monitoring the various conventions against torture including the 1948 Universal Declaration of Human Rights (UDHR), the 1966 International Covenant on Civil and Political Rights, the 1984 Convention against Torture, and the 1989 Convention on the Rights of the Child. The ICRC's role, via the 1949 Geneva Convention, is to have open access to POWs and civilians interned during international armed conflicts and civil wars.[5]

The most recent articulation of State's responsibilities in these matters is that provided by the UN's Convention against Torture and Other Cruel, Inhuman, or Degrading Treatment or Punishment (UN General Assembly Resolution 39/46) passed on December 10, 1984, and ratified on June 26, 1987. Some of the major points include Article 2 which states that there are no exceptional circumstances whatsoever may be invoked as a justification of torture, including a direct order from a superior officer or public authority. Article 3 prohibits the expulsion (refouler) or extradition of a person to another State where there are substantial grounds for believing they would be in danger of being subjected to torture while Article 4 mandates that signature States have criminal statutes both prohibiting and punishing those convicted of committing torture. Article 11 obliges States to systematically review its interrogation rules, instructions, methods, and practices as well as the custody and treatment of persons under arrest, detention, or incarceration within its jurisdiction. The United States signed the "Torture Convention" on April 18, 1988, and retracted on December 10, 2018, when allegations of torture emerged about U.S. acts during the Gulf Wars.[6]

America's Torturous History from the 1950s to Post-9/11/01

Despite the prominent role America played in the International War Tribunals following WWII, especially that of highlighting and criminalizing acts of torture and other crimes against humanity, it became involved in a clandestine era of terror in its fight against the perceived "communist threat." The seeds of this terrorism began immediately following WWII under the Truman administration (1945–1953) and accelerated under the Eisenhower (1953–1961) administration. With newly created Central Intelligence Administration (CIA), Allen Dulles initiated its clandestine operations in Latin America, pitting indigenous Indians and Mestizo peasants, those thought most prone to communist influence, against the dictators and U.S. business interest in these countries, giving the illusion of protecting the hemisphere from coming under Communist domination. Thus, "protecting the free world from Communism" became the mantra for the new era of the Monroe Doctrine in the Americas.

Invoking the Monroe Doctrine, the Eisenhower administration ruthlessly intervened in South and Central American affairs with deadly consequences that extended up until the Reagan administration (1981–1989). The CIA, America's secret police, was instrumental in training U.S. allies in the arts of torture, assassination, and terrorism. During the period 1952–1990, it is estimated that CIA-sponsored death squads killed hundreds of thousands in Latin America greatly contributing to the current unrest in these countries in the 21st century. The

1954 Guatemalan coup illustrates the CIA method. Guatemalan leader, General Jorge Ubico, a U.S.-sponsored dictator since 1930, who gave large landholdings to American United Fruit Company (UFCO), as well as housing U.S. military bases, was overthrown in 1944 during the country's first democratic elections. A number of events led to the U.S./CIA-led coup a decade later: President Juan Jose Arevalo established a minimum wage to the dismay of UFCO, which had long exploited the local workforce; while his successor, President Jacobo Arbenz, made additional social reforms including granting small landholdings to peasants (Mayan Indians/Mestizos) subsequently breaking up the large landholdings of UFCO. American capitalists soon pressured the U.S. government to intervene under the pretense of "fighting communism." Direct CIA action began with the coup of 1954 with a U.S.-sponsored paramilitary operation (PBHISTORY) that overthrew Arbenz installing a military dictator, Colonel Carlos Castillo Armas, as the U.S. and UFCO puppet. It was during this era that the Guatemalan government gave U.S. researchers free reign in conducting their sexually transmitted disease (STD) studies on the unsuspecting population. This continued until 1996 and only stopped due to media cries of genocide of the Mayan population.[7]

U.S. CIA-sponsored interventions continued through Latin America in Honduras, Panama, Bolivia, Columbia, Paraguay, Uruguay, Brazil, Costa Rica, El Salvador, Nicaragua, the Dominican Republic, and Haiti where death squads targeted mostly indigenous peasant populations and their traditional communal lifestyle. Much of this was hidden from the U.S. and world public until the Iran-Contra debacle under President Ronald Reagan. The U.S. Army School of the Americas (SOA), established in 1946 and headquartered in Panama until expelled in 1984, was the CIA's headquarters for Latin American interventions. It was then relocated to Fort Benning, Georgia. Here the CIA and U.S. Army manuals detailing torture techniques were developed. These techniques were used to train U.S.-backed militias notably in El Salvador, Guatemala, Ecuador, and Peru. The manuals described coercive interrogation techniques in detail torture techniques including psychological practices most likely to disorient captives such as early morning arrest, being blindfolded or hooded, stripped naked, being held incommunicado, subjected to sleep deprivation, and toilet deprivation—conducted in special windowless, soundproof, darkened interrogation rooms with extreme environmental variations. Waterboarding, sexual attacks and humiliation, mock executions, and other physical tortures such as being terrorized by attack dogs were taught as well, in addition to special terror death techniques (disappearances) like being thrown from helicopters in the presence of other prisoners.[8]

Despite leading the free world in the prohibitions against torture following WWII while directing the International Military Tribunals (IMTs) and preparing the language for the 1948 UDHR, America embarked on its own clandestine terrorists attacks on indigenous peasants in Latin America in support of business interests like United Fruit and mining and energy companies under the guise of "fighting" Communism and preserving Democracy in the hemisphere. These geopolitical interventions post-WWII continued until the early 21st century. Moreover, as they were not passive omissions of "looking the other way" relevant to serious human rights violations, the CIA provided the blueprint and training for illegal torture. Once disclosed and declassified in 2004, the 1963 and 1983 CIA torture manuals provided incontrovertible evidence to the nature and extent of these programs. The 1963 manual, *KUBARK Counterintelligence Interrogation*, outlined the basic premise of clandestine operations including torture and assassinations. KUBARK was cryptonym for the CIA. Included in the manuals were descriptions on the use of abusive techniques including electric shock and how to engender fear via sensory deprivation and other psychological methods. The revised 1983 version, *Human Resources Exploitation Training Manual*, also included a chapter on coercive techniques including steps in inducing psychological regression (aka "Reverse Malsow").

The particulars of the techniques promoted in the 1983 version were publically disclosed by *The Baltimore Sun* in 1994 and its expose on the CIA methods employed by Honduran Battalion 3–16 death squads.[9]

The list of CIA influence goes beyond the Americas (Argentina, Bolivia, Brazil, Chile, Colombia, Dominican Republic, El Salvador, Guatemala, Haiti, Mexico, Nicaragua, Peru, Paraguay, Uruguay, and Venezuela) including Greece, Portugal, Spain, Turkey, Indonesia, the Philippines, South Korea, Iran, Saudi Arabia, Morocco, Tunisia, and South Vietnam. Special attention is paid to the latter, notably the *Phoenix Program*. Here, the CIA directed its clandestine operations in conjunction with American, Australian, and friendly South Vietnam forces in its efforts to neutralize civilian supporters of the Viet Ming/Viet Cong (VC) via torture and assassinations (targeted killings). The methods employed included rape, rape*murder, electric shock to genitals or tongue, waterboarding, and the "airplane"—being suspended on a hook midair,—and police dog attacks. Murders involved being dropped from helicopters and inserting dowels into the ear canal into the brain. These techniques were administered to both men and women. It is estimated that in addition to some 26,000 noncombat deaths over three times that number were also subjected to torture. When forced to discontinue direct American military (U.S. Army and U.S. Marine Corps [USMC]) involvement, the CIA merely transferred the operations to the Vietnamese as Plan F-6. Ironically, these operations were classified as pacification methods designed to win over the Vietnamese populace.[10]

The Continued Use of Torture—The Gulf War Era

The post-Vietnam era conflicts included the first Gulf War, "Operation Desert Storm" (1991), following Iraq's attempt to incorporate Kuwait into its national boundaries. This was a short encounter under the George H.W. Bush administration (1989–1993). George H.W. Bush was also president during the early stages of the Bosnian war. Although the Gulf War was considered a success, it was not enough to get him a second term as president. His successor, William (Bill) Clinton (1993–2001), was instrumental in getting the United States more involved in the proxy, Yugoslavian civil wars (1991–1999) which included both the Bosnian war (1991–1995) and the Serbian/Kosovo conflict (1991–2001). Human rights abuses were alleged during both the first Bush administration and the Clinton administration.

The torture issue intensified following the horrific terrorist attacks of September 11, 2001. The chaos and pervasive fears of more attacks led to extra-legal actions directed toward the "outsiders" perceived responsible for the attacks. Even then geopolitics played a significant role in generating a convenient hated out-group—anti-Western culture, radical Islamic jihadists. Like in previous conflicts, the public was fed a selective list of potential enemies, conveniently downplaying the significance of the Saudi government in the attacks while drawing attention only to the main perpetrator, Al Qaeda, and its leader, Osama Bin Laden. Furthermore, the George W. Bush administration used the fear and fervor surrounding the 9/11/01 attacks to misdirect military aggression toward Saddam Hussein and Iraq which had nothing to do with the attacks. It was within this context and under these circumstances that America embarked on its insidious path toward gross human rights violations and its reintroduction of torture techniques it once condemned when used by others. The consequences of America's misguided actions in Iraq and Afghanistan ignited civil and proxy wars whose consequences are still being felt two decades later. The atmosphere for vindictive retribution in intergroup conflicts, like that of the Gulf Wars, is exacerbated when each side dehumanizes and demonizes the other. In retrospect, it is apparent that President George W. Bush faulty accused Saddam Hussein as having weapons of mass destruction as a pretext for the costly and destructive destruction of Iraq's society. The real reason was an excuse for a "punitive expedition" like President Wilson directed against Pancho Villa during the Mexican Revolution. Bush's reason was in response to Saddam Hussein's alleged threats made against his father, President George H.W. Bush, for initiating the first Gulf War in 1991. Reciprocal animosities increase proportionately to the degree of race/ethnic/cultural and sectarian differences hence setting the stage for fierce retribution under the guise of protecting one's group from the alien enemy. It is within these circumstances that the anti-Islamic versus anti-Western culture abuses occurred, including the political justification for human rights abuses including torture.

Critical to this process was establishing legal justifications for denying "enemy combatants," regardless if they were from Afghanistan or Iraq, due process under either U.S. or international laws. The foundation for the Bush torture mandate stems from the 1999 federal court decision stating the Fifth Amendment. The Fifth Amendment provides Grand Jury protection and review of the charges against a defendant:

> No person shall be held to answer for a capital, or otherwise infamous crime, unless on a presentment or indictment of a Grand Jury, except in cases arising in the land or naval forces, or in the Militia, when in actual service in time of War or public danger; nor shall any person be subject for the same offence to be twice put in jeopardy of life or limb; nor shall be compelled in any criminal case to be a witness against himself, no be deprived of life, liberty, or property, without due process of law; nor shall private property be taken for public use, without just compensation.[11]

Perhaps the most recognized element of the Fifth Amendment is the right against self-incrimination, "taking the Fifth." Another critical element is the right to due process which is reinforced by the 14th Amendment for U.S. citizens. An equally salient point is that of *habeas corpus*—allowing a prisoner to challenge his/her imprisonment in court. This is part of First Amendment. Accordingly, habeas corpus cannot be suspended except in extreme circumstances such as war where the public is in danger. Torture is also addressed by the Eighth Amendment which prohibits "cruel and unusual punishments."

The U.S. Military has its own judicial system, the Uniform Code of Military Justice (UCMJ), along with an appellant section—Courts of Appeals for the Armed Forces. In 1951, during the Korean Conflict, the UCMJ was expanded to include the Court of Appeals for the Armed Forces which consisted of a bench of five civilian judges. Accordingly, Article 36 allows for the U.S. president to prescribe rules and procedures for the UCMJ, whereas Articles 16–21 (chapter IV) specifies the UCMJ jurisdictional authority while Articles 30–35 (chapter VI) specifies pretrial procedures. About the same time (1950), the U.S. Supreme Court (USSC) ruled in *Johnson v. Eisentrager*, that captured enemy soldiers, not U.S. citizens, could not challenge habeas corpus detention within U.S. courts following a UCMJ conviction (court martial). In 1953, in *Burns v. Wilson*, the USSC allowed for UCMJ court martial appeals for soldiers who were U.S. citizens. Following the controversy of holding "enemy combatants" at the U.S. Naval base in Guantanamo, Cuba (GITMO), the USSC ruled in 2004, in *Rasul v. Bush*, that foreign nationals held at GITMO, or similar sites outside the United States, could petition the U.S. federal courts regarding the nature of their detention via habeas corpus appeals. In order to avoid allegations of violating the Geneva Convention dictates regarding POWs, the U.S. Congress passed and President George W. Bush signed Military Commissions Act (MCA) on October 7, 2006, establishing rules for adjudicating what the U.S. Department of Defense (DOD) signified as "unlawful enemy combatants" versus "lawful enemy combatants." However, the DOD and CIA's record on psychological warfare extends to the Korean

Conflict when the U.S. Military established its "Human Resources Research Organization," with active involvement of the American Psychological Association (APA).[12]

This complex legal maneuvering involvement of the interfacing of U.S. civilian and military justice set the stage for reintroducing and legitimizing torture during the Gulf War era and the role the APA played in this clandestine charade.

The deliberate mislabeling of POWs as criminals in order to justify cruel and unusual treatment did not originate with the George W. Bush administration. It was during the Woodrow Wilson administration (1913–1924) that the template for such ex-judicious treatment was initiated. Wilson's influence in the Mexican Revolution (1911–1917), notably his support for the Carranza forces in the civil war and providing temporary safe haven for Carranza's troops when pursued by General Pancho Villa, General of the oppositions northern army, led to Villas infamous cross-border raid on Columbus, New Mexico, on March 9, 1916—only the second time the U.S. mainland has been attacked by a foreign force (War of 1812 was the first). On that day, Villa accompanied by 485 troops conducted an early morning raid on the 13th U.S. Cavalry at Camp Furlong near Columbus, New Mexico. The raid had a dramatic effect on U.S./Mexican relations due to the audacity of the act even if it resulted in only 18 U.S. casualties (ten soldiers; eight civilians).[13]

Emotions ran high following General Villa's raid resulting in a rash of revenge killings of those of Mexican descent along the borderlands as the U.S. Army engaged in a hot pursuit of Villa's forces. President Wilson then made the unilateral decision for his "Punitive Expedition" into Mexico in pursuit of General Villa. The 11-month Punitive Expedition consisted of a force of 12,000 Army and National Guard troops led by Brigadier General John J. (Black Jack) Pershing. The punitive expedition brought considerable hardships to Mexicans already reeling from the devastations of their civil war. U.S. forces also clashed with Carranza's forces nearly leading to a full-fledged war with Mexico leading to passage of the National Defense Act in June 1916, authorizing the doubling of the size of the U.S. Army and authorizing the president to federalize the National Guard. While never capturing Villa, this action inadvertently prepared America for its entry into World War I (WWI) where General Pershing led the U.S. Expeditionary Forces.[14]

Not so well documented was the treatment of the Villista POWs. In order to provide a positive spin on the Punitive Expedition, the Wilson administration portrayed General Villa and his followers as "bandits" thereby attempting to exclude them from the 1907 Hague Convention concerning the laws and customs of war on land. In addition to the summary executions immediately following the Columbus raid and the subsequent 11-month Punitive Expedition (cut short by America's entry into WWI), 19 POWs caught by Pershing's troops in Mexico were charged with murder and tried in civilian courts where six were hanged. Those who were spared the death sentence in federal courts and served their prison term were soon rearrested by the Luna County, New Mexico, sheriff and again charged with murder and sentenced to additional terms in the state prison in blatant violation of the U.S. constitutional guarantee against double jeopardy. Thus, the process of labeling enemies opposed to U.S. interest and interventions in the Americas as being "bandits" as against legitimate military forces continued during the Monroe Doctrine/ Manifest Destiny era of clandestine operations in Latin America up until and including the Reagan Administration.[15]

Psychologists and Torture

The role of psychologists in establishing torture techniques during the George W. Bush administration following the 9/11/01 terrorist attacks was disclosed by Jane Mayer in a 2005 article in the *New Yorker* and discussed in detail in her 2008 book, *The Dark Side.* Mayer exposed the role of psychological consultants to the CIA's "Behavioral Science Consultation Team." Following the tradition of colleagues who assisted the DOD and the CIA during Operation Condor, and the Phoenix program, psychologist was again employed by the CIA in the post-9/11/01 era. Two licensed psychologists, Drs James Mitchell and Bruce Jessen, played a major role in redefining torture for the CIA. They and other contract psychologists devised "mind control" methods in order to break down human resistance in an adaptation of Martin Seligman's "learned helplessness theory," thereby deliberately creating psychological ambiguity fostering debility, dependency, and dread. Ostensibly, these methods were justified in order to obtain critical information relevant to future terrorist attacks, while a more compelling justification was that of psychological torture and retributive punishment. The psychologists also devised a training protocol in order for U.S. forces to resist similar techniques. This was the SERE program—"Survival, Evasion, Resistance and Escape." Incredibly, these psychologists aided and abetted torture with the blessings of the APA which secretly collaborated with the Bush administration in providing legal and ethical justifications for these gross human rights abuses.[16]

Once legitimized by both lawyer and psychologist, the George W. Bush embarked on a horror show of human rights abuses directed toward so-called "enemy combatants" which comprised of Muslim out-groups. These abuses included waterboarding, hooding, contorted stress positions, deafening noises, sexual humiliation, subjection to extreme heat or cold, coffin-like boxes, rectal rehydration, threats, etc. Death resulting from these abuses were often classified as suicides. These abuses and deaths occurred at the Guantanamo Base in Cuba and outsourced to numerous clandestine secret detention sites ("black sites") in 28 countries and on floating prison ships. The American public and the world became aware of the nature of these abuses when abuses at the U.S.-run prison at Abu Ghraib, Iraq, were exposed. Unfortunately, the true nature and extent of these abuses since the CIA was allowed to destroy all videotape evidence. Ironically, Gina Cheri Walker Haspel, the Director of the CIA since 2008—the first woman to hold that position—was complicit in the destruction of 92 interrogation videotapes while serving as Acting Director of the CIA's clandestine services. Hence, both the Obama (2009–2017) and Trump (2017–) administrations conspired to obviate evidence of these abuses. And a major player in the torture scandal, Dr. Susan Brandon, a research psychologist at Yale University, continued to advise both the George W. Bush and Obama administrations in her capacity as program officer at the U.S. National Institutes of Health (NIH) and as a "senior scientist" with the APA. As co-founder of SyncScience LLC, Brandon continues to profit from these positions.[17]

Brandon was instrumental in endorsing the two Air Force clinical psychologist, Drs James Mitchel (aka, Hammond Dunbar) and Bruce Jessen (aka, Grayson Swigert) and their torture enterprise, "Mitchell Jessen and Associates" to the CIA and the subsequent involvement of the APA in these activities and their cover-up. Another noted psychologist with Ivy League connection and government service, Dr. Norman B. Anderson, on the faculty of Harvard University's School of Public Health and former associate Director of NIH, and member of the National Academy of Sciences, was serving as the first Black CEO of the APA. He inherited this position from Raymond D. Fowler who became the APA's first CEO following his tenure as the APA's 97th president (1988) serving from 1989 until 2003. Dr. Anderson then served from 2003 until his forced retirement in 2015. Parallels exist between the Tuskegee Syphilis Study (1932–1972) and the CIA's clandestine psychological warfare programs. Both involved high-status academics who held prestigious positions within the federal government health apparatus who, in turn, were able to coop others in participating in what were obviously gross ethnic violations in the name of government-sponsored programs. This complicity earned numerous psychologist, including APA presidents, awards such as the "APA Distinguished Scientific Contribution Award," as well as considerable wealth.[18]

Once the "torture memos" were publically disclosed both the American Psychiatric Association (ApA) and the American Medical Association (AMA) in 2006 determined that any direct participation in interrogations constituted a serious ethical violation and therefore forbidden. The APA, on the other hand, began its whitewash of its involvement in "torturegate."[19] In June 2005, the APA disseminated its "Report of the APA Presidential Task Force on Psychological Ethics and National Security (PENS)." This "consensus report" outlined 12 statements concerning psychologists' "Ethical Obligations in National Security-Related Work":

1. Psychologists do not engage in, direct, support, facilitate, or offer training in torture or other cruel, inhuman, or degrading treatment.
2. Psychologists are alert to acts of torture and other cruel, inhuman, or degrading treatment and have an ethical responsibility to report these acts to the appropriate authorities (Ethical Standard 3.04, Avoiding Harm).
3. Psychologists who serve in the role of supporting an interrogation do not use health care related information from an individual's medical record to the detriment of the individual's safety and well-being (Ethical Standards 3.04, Avoiding Harm; 3.08, Exploitative Relationships).
4. Psychologists do not engage in behaviors that violate the laws of the United States, although psychologists may refuse for ethical reasons to follow laws or offers that are unjust or that violate basic principles of human rights (Ethical Standard 1.02).
5. Psychologists are aware of and clarify their role in situations where the nature of their professional identity and professional function may be ambiguous (Ethical Standards 3.07, Third Party Requests for Services; 3.11, Psychological Services Delivery to or Through Organizations; 3.09, Cooperating with Other Professionals).
6. Psychologists are sensitive to the problem inherent in mixing potentially inconsistent roles such as health care provider and consultant to an interrogation and refrain from engaging in such multiple relationships (Ethical Standard 3.05, Multiple Relationships).
7. Psychologists may serve in various national security-related roles, such as a consultant to an interrogation, in a manner that is consistent with the Ethical Code, and when doing so psychologists are mindful of factors unique to these roles and contexts that require special ethical consideration (Ethical Standards 1.01, Misuse of Psychologist' Work; 3.08, Exploitative Relationships; 2.01, Boundaries of Competence; 3.01, Unfair Discrimination; 3.04, Avoiding Harm).
8. Psychologists who consult on interrogation techniques are mindful that the individual being interrogated may not have been engaged in untoward behavior and may not have information of interests to the interrogator (Ethical Standards 2.01, Boundaries of Competence; 2.03, Maintaining Competence; 3.01, Unfair Discrimination).
9. Psychologists make clear the limits of confidentiality (Ethical Standards 4.02, Discussing the Limits of Confidentiality; 4.01, Maintaining Confidentiality; 4.04, Minimizing Intrusions on Privacy; 3.01, Informed Consent).
10. Psychologists are aware of and do not act beyond their competencies, except in unusual circumstances, such as set forth in the Ethics Code (Ethical Standards 2.02, Providing Services in Emergencies; 2.01, Boundaries of Competence; 2.04, Bases for Scientific and Professional Judgments; 9.01, Bases for Assessments).

11. Psychologists clarify for themselves the identity of their client and retain ethical obligations to individuals who are not their clients (Ethical Standards 3.04, Avoiding Harm; 3.08, Exploitative Relationships).
12. Psychologists consult when they are facing difficult ethical dilemmas (Ethical Standard 4.06, Consultations).[20]

Critics of the PENS Report noted that the leadership at the APA at the time forged its report so as to appease the DOD and the CIA so as to continue receiving lucrative grants and contracts. This was accomplished by stacking the Task Force with DOD sympathizers and insiders with the aid of Pentagon influence producing a report that purportedly justified the use of psychologists in teaching and implementing torture and other human rights violations, such as forced feedings, on those peoples defined as being hostile to the United States and denied access to UN human right protocols. Notably among those voicing opposition to the PENS Report was a group known as the "Coalition for an Ethical Psychology" (www.ethicalpsychology.org) which proposed, "A Resolution to Annul the APA's PENS Report:"

> That Council annul the American Psychological Association's (APA's) 2005 Presidential Report on Psychological Ethics and National Security (the "PENS Report").
>
> WHEREAS reports circulated as early as 2004 that psychologists acted as planners, consultants, researchers, and overseers to abusive and sometimes torturous interrogations at Guantanamo Bay Detentions Center, Bagram Air Base, and CIA "black sites";
>
> WHEREAS the PENS Task Force ignored the Board mandate to inquire into the specific public reports of psychologist involvement in abusive interrogations at Guantanamo, the CIA's secret prisons, and elsewhere, in spite of the fact that the Task Force contained several members with direct knowledge of the torture and other abusive interrogations conducted or aided by psychologists;
>
> WHEREAS the PENS Report nevertheless endorsed psychologists' involvement in interrogations of national security detainees as a means to ensure that they are safe, legal, ethical, and effective;
>
> WHEREAS six of the nine voting members of the PENS Task Force were on the payroll of the U.S. military and/or intelligence agencies, and several of them were drawn from chains of command accused of abuses under the purview of Task Force ethical guidance;
>
> WHEREAS the military members of the PENS Task Force required as a condition of their participation that the PENS Report be framed within U.S. law rather than international human rights law, even though APA is an accredited NGO to the United Nations;
>
> WHEREAS senior representatives from the APA Ethics Office, Public Affairs Office, Science Directorate, and Private Directorate were undisclosed participants in the weekend PENS Task Force meeting;
>
> WHEREAS some of these representatives engaged in high-level lobbying for Department of Defense (DoD) funding and had a vested interest in a PENS Report compatible with then current DoD policy;
>
> WHEREAS a significant conflict of interest existed for the Director of the APA Practice Directorate (who played a dominant role during the Task Force meetings) because his wife was an active duty, SERE-trained psychologist who served at Guantanamo; she was also responsible in part for developing the practice and training models for psychologists involved in detainee interrogations at Guantanamo;

WHEREAS the employment status of several Task Force members and others in attendance required or encouraged them to support psychologist participation in national security interrogations and to accommodate the Bush Administration's permissive legal definition of torture rather than the stricter definition of torture in international human rights law;

WHEREAS the Task Force and unacknowledged participants presumed, without introduced evidence, the military necessity of psychologist involvement in interrogation and detainee operations;

WHEREAS the PENS Task Force presumed that the current APA Ethics Code adequately addressed complex ethical issues associated with psychologists involvement in national security operations, that no new ethical standards were needed, and that national security concerns justified subordinating individual interest to government interest;

WHEREAS the PENS Task Force declined to consider the challenges in adapting the APA Ethics Code to operational psychologist working under military authority and military exigencies, including the difficult or impossibility of ethical monitoring of actions and of obtaining independent consultation in classified settings;

WHEREAS there was little or no consultation with psychologists from other specialties that would be affected by, and concerned about, the policy, and no subsequent period was provided for member feedback;

WHEREAS the PENS Task Force Chair designated two non-members of the Task Force—the Director of the Ethics Office and the Office of Public Affairs—as the sole spokespersons for the Task Force, and a highly unusual confidentiality agreement bound the Task Force members from discussing the proves or the Report with others;

WHEREAS official APA acceptance of the PENS Report departed from standard APA procedures in the following ways: the director of its Ethics Office was appointed as "rapporteur" and he produced the full draft report at the close of the two-and-a-half-day meeting; the Task Force members were given 24 hours to accept or reject the report; the APA Board of Directors invoked its emergency powers to endorse the PENS Report, preempting a standard review and vote by the Council of Representatives; and approval was not sought from the Policy and Planning Board, the Board of Professional Affairs, or the Board for Advancement of Psychology in the Public Interest;

WHEREAS the identities of the PENS Task Force members were not included in the Report, were not posted on the APA's website, and were withheld from members of the APA and members of the press requesting them;

WHEREAS these processes were far outside the norms of transparency, independence, and deliberation for similar task forces established by the APA and by other professional associations;

WHEREAS two voting members of the Task Force not employed by national security agencies, upon further reflection after the pressured weekend meeting, rejected the PENS Report and called for its annulment, with one resigning from the Task Force in protest;

WHEREAS the PENS Report has been cited routinely in Behavioral Science Consultant policy memos as supporting psychologists' involvement in detention, interrogation, and debriefing operations, including in the assessment and exploitation of individual detainee "vulnerabilities" for intelligence purposes;

WHEREAS the PENS Report is being used to support the promotion of "operational psychology"—which includes applications of psychology to direct harm to those identified as potential adversaries—as an official area of specialization for psychologists;

WHEREAS the PENS Report is repeatedly cited as a resource for ethical decision-making in the APA Ethics Committee's recent "casebook" on National Security Commentary;

WHEREAS the PENS Report has contributed to significant harm to vulnerable populations by supporting policies that permit abusive treatment; has badly damaged the reputation of the profession of psychology; has diminished the APA's commitment to advance psychology "as a means of promoting health, education and human welfare"; has compromised the integrity of the relationship between professional psychology and the security sector; and according to some senior interrogators and intelligence professionals, has undermined national security;

WHEREAS the PENS Task Force meeting was purported to be the one forum where the ethics of psychologist involvement in problematic national security activities were discussed and resolved, yet Task Force members failed to engage in any substantive dialogue about psychological ethics and national security;

THEREFORE BE IT RESOLVED that the APA's Report of the Presidential Task Force on Psychological Ethics and National Security (PENS Report) is hereby annulled (July 26, 2112).[21]

The Coalition for an Ethical Psychology was established, by concerned psychologists such as Stephen Soldz, Roy Eidelson, and Steven Reisner, as a rapid response to the PENS Report. The Coalition's resolution was effectively ignored and stonewalled until James Risen's book, *Pay any Price*, implicated the APA in the Bush administrations torture activities. This expose finally forced the APA to take action doing so at the Annual APA conference held in Toronto, Canada, in August 2015. A major outcome was the hiring of the law firm, Sidney Austin, with David H. Hoffman conducting an independent review of the PENS Report. In a nutshell, Hoffman's report outlined the clandestine role the APA and member psychologists, like James Mitchell and Bruce Jessen, played in justifying human rights abuses as meeting APA-Ethical Standards conducted by the DOD and the CIA. The Hoffman report also highlighted the APA's elaborate cover-up in this matter.[22] Lawsuits and countersuits abounded but eventually the desired outcome was achieved—a strengthening of the APA Ethics to follow international human rights standards. Following the submission of the Hoffman report and the pending "retirement" of Norman Anderson as CEO, the membership overwhelmingly passed Resolution 23B at the 123rd annual convention in Toronto, Canada, that called for the revocation of APA members who violate international law that involve unlawful interrogations. Now APA policies fall in line with that of the ApA and the AMA by explicitly prohibiting psychologists from participating in interrogations that go against the dictates of the Geneva Conventions and the UN Convention against Torture. The AMA's doctrine is as follows:

The *Code* offers specific policy regarding what physicians should and should not do in situations involving torture or coercive interrogation. With regard to torture, several key principles from Opinion E-2.067 must be observed:

- Physicians must oppose and must not participate in torture for any reason. Participation in torture includes, but is not limited to, providing or withholding any services, substances or knowledge to facilitate the practice of torture. Physicians must not be present when torture is used or threatened.
- Physicians should only treat individuals when it is in the patient's interest, not to verify health so that torture can begin or continue.

- Physicians should help provide support for victims of torture and whenever possible strive to change situations in which torture is practiced or the potential for torture is great.

The opinion also notes that physicians who follow their calling as healers in treating torture victims should not be persecuted.

For interrogation, physicians must avoid being involved in anything that uses coercion (defined as "threatening or causing harm through physical injury or mental suffering"). Physicians have five ethical obligations under Opinion E-2.068:

- Physicians should only perform physical and mental assessments of detainees to determine the need for and to provide medical care. When doing so, physicians must disclose the extent to which others have access to information included in medical records. Treatment must never be conditional on a patient's participation in an interrogation.
- Physicians must neither conduct nor directly participate in an interrogation. Being involved in interrogation undermines the physician's role as healer and thereby erodes trust in the individual physician and in the medical profession.
- Physicians must not monitor interrogations with the intention of intervening in the process. This constitutes direct participation in interrogation.
- Physicians should not participate in developing effective interrogation strategies except for general training purposes. These strategies must not threaten or cause physical injury or mental suffering and must be humane and respect the rights of individuals.
- Physicians must report their observations to the appropriate **authorities** if they have reason to believe that interrogations are coercive. If those authorities are aware of coercive interrogations but have not intervened, physicians are ethically obligated to report the offenses to independent authorities that have the power to investigate or adjudicate such allegations.

"We firmly believe that U.S. policies on detainee treatment must comport with the AMA's *Code of Medical Ethics* and the World Medical Association's Declaration of Tokyo, which forcefully state medicine's opposition to torture or coercive interrogation and prohibit physician participation in such activities," AMA President Robert M. Wah, MD, said.

"The AMA will continue to advocate that no doctor is asked to go against the ethics of the profession," Dr. Wah said.

Archived articles in the AMA's online ethics journal *Virtual Mentor* further explore the issue of physician obligations concerning torture and interrogations. Insights from physicians and other experts in the field include:

- The role of physicians in interrogations. Physicians have recognized responsibilities to patients and society. This article explores the question of whether honoring the societal responsibility allows a physician to participate in interrogation and if so, to what extent.
- Torture and human rights. Involvement in torture—before, during and even afterward—puts physicians in morally compromised positions, no matter whether civil, military or judicial systems have approved it. This article discusses how physicians in the military, especially those called on to care for prisoners, should heed the counsel of their professional organizations and avoid all complicity with torture.[23]

Human Rights violations currently are heard internationally by the ICC. The International Court of Justice, the carryover from the League of Nations, became the ICC. The Rome Statute of the

ICC led to the establishment of the ICC in 2002 as a permanent international court. Having played a major role in the establishment of the international courts adjudication process in the post-WWII IMTs and the Clinton administration's (1993–2001) prominent role in the Bosnian and Kosovo wars, President Clinton signed the Rome Statute in 2000 as a token measure while not submitting it for needed Senate ratification.

Clinton's successor, President George W. Bush (2001–2009), flatly refused to join the ICC mainly due to abuses of Iraqi POWs during the Second Gulf War. The Obama administration (2009–2017) merely signed on with "observer" status. In 2002, the U.S. Bush administration withdrew from supporting the ICC even though President Clinton signed the United States up in 2000. U.S. support was crucial for the International Criminal Tribunal-Yugoslavia (ICTY) adjudication of war crimes during the Balkan Wars; however, deliberate violations of the Geneva Convention and UN proscriptions against torture and illegal detentions associated with the wars in Iraq and Afghanistan set the stage for the U.S. exit from international justice jurisdiction. To further distant the United States from the rest of the world, the Trump administration leveled sanctions against ICC prosecutors investigating alleged human rights abused and other war crimes conducted by Americans in Afghanistan.

The U.S. "Torture" issue raises questions concerning the "professional suitability" of psychologists, notably those licensed within the clinical and forensic fields. This is different from academic suitability where grade point averages (GPA) and test scores are used to determine acceptance into clinical and/or legal practice. Professional suitability addresses the more visceral components of our persona—our intrinsic prejudices and biases—which all of us inherent from our socialization and enculturation. Psychologist Stanley Milgram and Philip Zimbardo alluded to the human potential for sadistic behaviors under certain circumstances especially situations where these behaviors are condoned and justified as being for the greater good. This atmosphere of chaos and danger challenges the status quo challenging our moral compass leading to risky behaviors and enhanced status. The latter refers to the *vicarious warrior syndrome*, a component gleaned from Zimbardo's *Lucifer Effect* on how good people turn evil. The *vicarious warriors* refer to professionals whose noncombat status and ego, like military psychologist, is greatly enhanced by their involvement in seemingly dangerous and quasi-legal behaviors that are rewarded by higher echelon officials. Clinical psychologists, like law enforcement personnel, need to be tested for their professional suitability by using instruments that attempt to measure their degree of biases and prejudices: instruments like the F-Scale (Fascist) and the Locus of Control for their degrees of intolerance for "others."[24]

Notes

1 *Death.* San Francisco, CA: W.H. Freeman.
2 *Ibid.*; Selye, H. 1976. *The Stress of Life.* New York, NY: McGraw-Hill; Selye, H. 1976. *Stress in Health and Disease.* Boston, MA: Butterworth.
3 See *Law of War Manual.* 2016. Washington, DC: United States Department of Defense.
4 See ICRC. *Prohibition and Punishment of Torture and Other Forms of Ill-treatment,* Advisory Service on International Humanitarian Law. www.icrc.org/customary-ihl/eng/docs/home.
5 *Ibid.*
6 See UN. *Convention against Torture and Other Cruel, Inhuman or Degrading Treatment or Punishment* (Torture Convention). New York, NY: United Nations Treaty Series, Vol. 1465, p. 85. www.refworld.org/docoid/.
7 See Cullather, N. 1999. *Secret History: The CIA's Classified Account of Its Operations in Guatemala, 1952–1954.* Palo Alto, CA: Stanford University Press; Immerman, R.H. 1982. *The CIA in Guatemala: The*

Foreign Policy of Intervention. Austin, TX: University of Texas Press; Kinzer, S., & Schlesinger, S. 1999. *Bitter Fruit: The Story of the American Coup in Guatemala*. Cambridge, MA: Harvard University Press.

8 See Lesley, G. 2004. *The School of the Americas: Military Training and Political Violence in the Americas*. Durham, NC: Duke University Press.

9 See, Lesley, op. cit. 8; CIA, *KUBARK Counterintelligence Interrogation, July 1963* and *Human Resource Exploitation Training Manual-1983*. Washington, DC: National Security Archive; *Fact Sheet Concerning Training Manuals Containing Materials Inconsistent with U.S. Policy from the Office of the Assistant Secretary of Defense/Public Affairs Office*. www.gwu.edu/-nsarchiv/nsa/archive/news/dodmans.htm.

10 See Tirman, J. 2011. *The Deaths of Others: The Fate of Civilians in America's Wars*. New York, NY: Oxford University Press; Valentine, D. 2014. *The Phoenix Program: America's Use of Terror in Vietnam*. Forbidden Bookshelf; Cook, J.L. 1973. *The Advisor: The Phoenix Program in Vietnam*. Philadelphia, PA: Dorrance & Company; Chomsky, N., & Herman, E.S. 1973. *Counter-Revolutionary Violence: Bloodbaths in Fact & Propaganda*. Andover, MA: Warner Modular Publications.

11 See *The CONSTITUTION of the UNITED STATES OF AMERICA, Amendment V.*

12 See *Uniform Code of Military Justice* 1951. United States Code, Title 10 (UCMJ); *Johnson v. Eisentrager* 399 U.S. 763 (1950); *Burns v. Wilson* 346 U.S. 137 (1953); *Rasul v. Bush,* 542 U.S. 466 (2004); Murphy, S.D. 2001. *Military Commissions Act (MCA)*. Public Law 109-366. U.S. Statutes at Large 120 stat. 2600 (October 2006); Application of Fifth Amendment to overseas torture of alien. *American Journal of International Law,* Vol. 95 (3), pp. 641–643.

13 See Thompkins, F. 1934. *Chasing Villa: The Last Campaign of the U.S. Cavalry*. Harrisburg, PA: Military Service Publishing Company; Clendenen, C.C. 1961. *The United States and Pancho Villa: A Study in Unconventional Diplomacy*. Ithaca, NY: American Historical Association. Cornell University Press.

14 *Ibid.*

15 See Hurst, J.W. 2000. *The Villista Prisoners of 1916–1917*. Las Cruces, NM: Yucca Tree Press.

16 See Mayer, J. 2008. *The Inside Story of How the War on Terror Turned into a War on American Ideals*. New York, NY: Doubleday.

17 See Cole, D. 2013. *The Torture Memos: Rationalizing the Unthinkable*. New York, NY: The New Press.

18 *Ibid.*

19 See Risen, J. 2014. *Pay Any Price: Greed, Power, and Endless War*. Boston, MA: Houghton, Mifflin Harcourt.

20 Arrigo, J.M., & Wessells, M. June 2005. *Report of the American Psychological Association Presidential Task Force on Psychological Ethics and National Security*. Washington, DC: American Psychological Association.

21 See *Coalition for an Ethical Psychology: Human Rights, Ethics, Social Justice: A Resolution to Annul the APA's PENS Report*. July 2012. www.ethicalpsychology.org.

22 See Hoffman, D., et al. July 2, 2015. *The Hoffman Report: The Investigation into the American Psychological Association (APA)*. Independent Review Relating to APA Ethics Guidelines, National Security Interrogations, and Torture. Chicago, IL: Sidley Austin, LLC.

23 Wah, R.M. (AMA President). December 12, 2014. *AMA Ethics: Torture, Coercive Interrogations and Physicians*. Washington, DC: American Medical Association.

24 See Milgram, S. 1974. *Obedience to Authority*. New York, NY: Harper & Row; Zimbardo, P. 2008. *The Lucifer Effect: How Good People Turn Evil*. New York, NY: Random House.

7

ABUSE OF PRIVILEGE

Social Stratification and Elitism

Most societies historically, and today, are stratified by caste, class, and/or gender. Those residing at the apex of the hierarchy are afforded the greatest status and privilege. This is human nature. It does not, in itself, connote abuse per se in that a majority of the group's membership needs to concur with the status quo for its continuation. Elite status follows various social scenarios with some following a sectarian ordination while others use royal or other forms of inheritance and some follow a political route. As stated earlier in Chapter 1, this need for social structure is linked to the relative structure of societies and the human need for psychological boundary maintenance—that is the need to know "our place" vis-à-vis others within our group and in relations to "other" groups.

Like Philip Zimbardo but over a century earlier, Emile Durkheim, the noted French existential sociologist, articulated the significance of our "sense of self" being linked to a group from which we glean our identity. Durkheim's "Lucifer Effect" gave a broader perspective on group dynamics and human identity where he noted that even in a perfect saintly society, "deviance" would exist/created for the sake of defining the group's social stratification and acceptable boundaries that articulate the group's existence at any given time. Moreover, Durkheim saw role conflict and status marginality being linked to a person's degree of integration into the society or group. Hence, our group-engendered status/role integration, that is, "our place in society or the group," often competes with the formal rules and expectations demanded by those governing the society of which we hold membership. Our integration into the group greatly influences both our psyche and our behaviors. Chaos can engender normlessness (anomie) and a sense of loss and vulnerability. Within this scenario, where group members are assigned to various strata within society, symbiotic relationships are formed. In many instances, these relationships are defined by age, gender, and race/ethnic/tribal identity. Clearly, inter-strata abuses are more likely to occur within caste systems where people are strictly confined to their strata which are often defined by physical characteristics such as gender or race/ethnicity. America established its own aristocracy during the colonial era and its moral justification for a power elite based on White supremacy.[1]

DOI: 10.4324/9781003224426-7

Institutionalized and Systemic Sexism

A common milieu for exploitation, notably sexual exploitation (sexploitation), exists when someone in a trusted, privileged position exploits the vulnerabilities of those under their care. This was noted in the previous discussions relevant to informed consent and duty to warn and report. Sex abuse of minors by clergy or Boy Scout leaders and police harassment of people of color are prime examples of these types of abuse. The fact that these abuses occur under many social circumstances where those in power abuse subordinates became widely disseminated through the *#Me Too Movement*. Tarana Burke is credited in starting the *#Me Too Movement* in 2006 via social media by publicizing sexual abuse and sexual harassment on her Myspace account. The movement gained widespread attention leading to the firing of high-status males in numerous occupations.

Most notably were the convictions and incarceration of well-known celebrities Bill Cosby and Harvey Weinstein. Bill Cosby who portrayed a compassionate father and husband on his popular TV show, "The Cosby Show" from 1984 to 1992 was accused by over 60 women of sexual abuse including drug-facilitated sexual assault. He was convicted and sentenced to 3–10 years in September 2018 and remains incarcerated at this time. Harvey Weinstein, Academy Award-winning producer, epitomized the "casting couch" stereotype with some 80 women leveled sexual abuse accusations against him. He was found guilty on five counts and sentenced to a 23-year sentence in February 2020. Both men tried to use the "its was consensual sex" defense adding that the alleged victims readily accepted "non-disclosure payment" in order to shield the accused from criminal liability, a process that implied "post-factor prostitution" on the part of the accusers. These convictions ended the long-held tradition of ignoring cries of sexual harassment by prominent men finally given credence to Brandeis University Professor Anita Hill's accusations of sexual harassment against Clarence Thomas. At the time, in 1991, Hill exposed herself to ridicule when testifying before the U.S. Senate at Thomas' Supreme Court confirmation hearings where she spoke of severe sexual harassment by Thomas when he was her supervisor at the U.S. Department of Education and on the Equal Employment Opportunity Commission. Despite her public accusations, Clarence Thomas was appointed as an Associate Justice to the U.S. Supreme Court serving in that capacity since 1991.

While much attention had been focused on race and class, gender biases emerged as the most prevalent and pervasive form of exploitation if only because it transcends class and race existing at all levels of society. Indeed, it can be said that "institutionalized and systemic gender bias" exists at every level of American society within and between social classes. The roots of America's male-dominated gender bias, and the methods of its perpetuations via education and class dynamics, extend to the colonial era its White Anglo-Saxon Protestant (WASP) males which dictated America's cast and class divides. The idea of paternalistic provision and protection for its women and children obviated abuses that occurred within this private domain, a phenomenon that transcribe race, ethnicity, and class. Historically, women often had little recourse in addressing physical and sexual abuse. In the United States, the 13th Amendment freed males, notably Blacks, from slavery but did not free women from involuntary servitude via marriage or other means of conscription. Technically, all males were enfranchised in 1865 according to the 13th Amendment while, in reality, this right was thwarted by Jim Crow law until the Civil Rights Movement a century later. Hence, White women were enfranchised in 1920 with passage of the 19th Amendment while women of color had to wait until the 1960s. American Indians, male or female, were not federally enfranchised until 1924. Equal Rights Amendment (ERA) calling for equal legal rights for women gained attention during the Civil Rights Movement of the 1960s and 1970s. The ERA was reintroduced by Representative Martha Griffiths in 1971 and was approved by the U.S. House of Representatives on October 12, 1971, and by the U.S. Senate on March 22, 1972, setting the stage for it being submitted to the state legislatures for ratification, as provided for in Article V of the U.S. Constitution. Congress set a ratification deadline of March 22, 1979, for the state legislatures to consider the ERA. The amendment did not receive the necessary 38 state ratifications by the deadline and five states subsequently reversed its legislative support while others approved it beyond the 1979 deadline leaving the Amendment currently in limbo. The ERA is designed to place women on an equal economic level as men regarding equal pay for similar jobs.

The blight of sex discrimination is worse for enslaved women. Some of the abuse has disproportionately affected women of color. This was discussed previously in this book with the slew of Chinese exclusion acts of the late 19th-century labeling females as "prostitutes" and the involuntary sterilization of Black, Metizo Hispanics, and American Indians by White-dominated Jim Crow states and the federal government (Indian Country) during the Eugenics era that lasted until the 1970s. The battle over a woman's right to self-determination continues to the present in the constant legal challenges to the 1973 U.S. Supreme Court decision, *Roe v. Wade* regarding abortion.[2]

The 1970s were for the most part the transformation decade for ethics and human rights and attention toward institutional racism in America. In the early 1970s, I conducted a study on race and incarceration in North Carolina during the time of the U.S. Supreme Court's 1972 decision, *Furman v. Georgia*, finding America's death sentence as unconstitutional as practiced. North Carolina was among those states with a highly discriminatory death sentence at the time of the moratorium (capital punishment was reinstated in 1976 following the strict USSC guidelines). My study looked at the maximum security prison and the Correctional Center for Women. My summary of the situation in the 1970s is as follows:

> Using the North Carolina Correctional system in general, and specifically two correctional institutions as an example, some serious inconsistencies are illuminated. It is apparent that the justice ideals of equal justice seem instead to be noticeably selective, especially along class, race and sex lines. Incarceration seems heavily influenced by these three variables in that there is a greater chance for a person who is poor, Black, and male to be incarcerated in North Carolina prisons. The findings from this investigation clearly show that the majority of those incarcerated were Black, on the lower economic level, and male.
>
> … The women in prison reflect the same discriminatory patterns found among their male counterparts regarding class and race. This analysis indicates that Blacks and lower class females have an even higher percentage representation in the North Carolina correctional system that do black males, even though the latter accounts for the greatest number of incarcerated persons in the state.
>
> … It seems apparent that the same type of prisoners who populated the prisons and chain gangs in the early (post-Civil War) North Carolina's prison history still populate North Carolina prisons today … If this is so, then there is further reason to believe that the discriminatory justice as practiced earlier in history still exists. If the functions of America's judicial process do not facilitate or actualize its ideal mandate of equal justice, then what purpose does it serve and who benefits? A plausible answer focuses on the boundary-maintenance concept of relative justice and elitism. This perspective views justice and selective adjudication as being relative in that it is defined in line with the value system of those in control of society's main institutions, one that often is used to perpetuate the power differential between the "haves" and the "have nots."[3]

The civil rights and anti-war chaos of the 1960s and 1970s forced Americans to revisit its biased criminal justice system, one where institutionalized racism went well beyond the Jim Crow South. An innovative outgrowth of the 1968 Omnibus Crime Control and Safe Streets Act was the educational component of the Law Enforcement Assistance Administration (LEAA), the forum for the distribution of block grants to states as well as federal initiatives. A unique U.S. Department of Justice (DOJ) program was the "Education Project in Criminal Justice" established at the State University of New York (SUNY-A) college of criminal justice in 1977–1978. The program was designed to develop a model minority criminal justice curriculum for college-level criminal justice programs nationwide. Toward this end, 20 "college instructors," representing minority (Blacks, Hispanics, Asians, and American Indians), were selected mainly from minority-serving colleges and universities. Thirteen (10 males; 3 females) of the 20 minority faculty were from Historically Black Colleges and Universities (HBCUs) in the South. The Black component was rounded out with two Hispanics (one of White Cuban descent and one of Chicano/Mexican descent), an Asian of Chinese, two White faculty, one teaching at a HBCU, a male of Arab descent, and me—representing American Indians.

Ostensibly, the manifest function of the SUNY-A program was to glean valuable insights from the "minority faculty," and it quickly became apparent that the real purpose (latent function) was to school the 20 participants in the White-elitists perspective of American justice. The "Major Professors" and their associates were White with one exception, a Black sociology professor from Pennsylvania State University. Marvin Wolfgang from the University of Pennsylvania, a main perpetrator of inherent Black criminality, was the main indoctrinator of this group. The condescending arrogance of Wolfgang and his cohorts with their attempt to put forth their agenda led to a revolt among the minority participants, myself included. More surprising to me was the internal debate among the three Black female faculty who chastised their male counterparts for their traditional, systemic male dominance and poor treatment of Black females in all aspects of Black lives. This was expressed as being "second-class" citizens within a second-class subculture. That aside, the SUNY-A program assessment noted the failure of this program, along with its false pretense of soliciting minority input. The program's outcome assessment states that: "the patronizing elitism of the Major Professors and their associates obviated the two-way communication necessary for a project like this to succeed." The program evaluators, the National Council of Black Lawyers, concurred with this assessment.[4]

A group suffering from serious abuses, mental, physical, and sexual is American Indian women especially those residing in federally protected Indian Country. Substance abuse fostered by an impoverished environment is a major mitigating factor in the high incident of abuse of Indian and Alaska Native women. Attention to Indian women came as a result of Congress passing the Violence Against Women Act (VAWA) in 1994 as part of Title IX of the U.S. Civil Rights Act. The subsequent findings of the Congressional probe into its own federal responsibilities in Indian County; it passed *Safety for Indian Women* in 2013 as a component of Title IX. Here, Congress found:

1. 1 out of every 3 Indian (including Alaska Native) women are raped in their lifetime;
2. Indian women experience 7 sexual assaults per 1,000, compared with 4 per 1,000 among Black Americans, 3 per 1,000 among Caucasians, 2 per 1,000 among Hispanic women, and 1 per 1,000 among Asian women;
3. Indian women experience the violent crime of battering at a rate of 23.2 per 1,000 compared with 8 per 1,000 among Caucasian women;
4. During the period 1979 through 1992, homicide was the third leading cause of death of Indian females aged 15 to34, and 75 percent were killed by family members or acquaintances;

5. Indian tribes require additional criminal justice and victim services resources to respond to violent assaults against women; and
6. The unique legal relationship of the United States to Indian tribes creates a Federal trust responsibility to assist tribal governments in safeguarding the lives of Indian women.[5]

The problem of abuse of Indigenous women in the United States, both on and off reservations (Indian Country), continues unabated. Added to this dilemma is the incredible number of missing and murdered American Indian/Alaska Native women and girls with over 5,700 reported as of 2016 and only 116 cases actively investigated. To address this problem, President Donald Trump (2017–2021) established an Indian Affairs Task Force on November 28, 2019, that comprises of both the U.S. DOJ and the U.S. Department of the Interior using federal law enforcement agencies including the Federal Bureau of Investigation (FBI) which has original jurisdiction over major crimes on federal lands including Indian Country.[6]

Education and Privilege: The Socialization of the Elite

Sociologists recognize that social status and role expectations are inculcated in both the family and educational settings. Social stratification is an important element of this process. The dynamics of both inclusion and exclusion need to be made evident throughout the society for social strata to be effective. Both the in-group and out-group members must know "their place" for the society to establish any semblance of boundary maintenance. Privilege, status, and control are all associated with effective socialization—with education being the major vehicle of dissemination of these critical factors. Essentially, it is our socialization that determines our "audience"—the group for which we perform and expect satisfactory feedback. In many societies, only its aristocracy allows its privileged classes access to high-status positions via its elite educational system.

Europe's aristocracy allowed only the privileged classes access to high-status positions via its elite "public" schools. Although aristocratic lineage did not transfer to America following the Revolutionary War, class and caste has always been part and parcel of U.S. culture with educational accessibility the primary vehicle for status enhancement. The privileged elite in America has always had access to prestigious schools, a type of entitlement that allows these peoples to remain at the helm of the capitalist economic and political system. Education in the original 13 British colonies originated as agents of sectarian indoctrination. Massachusetts, the colony that led the colonies in educational endeavors, was clearly a theocracy with little tolerance for other epistemological methodologies. While the Pilgrims came to the New World ostensibly to escape religious persecution, they, in fact, were a closed intolerant society with little tolerance for other sectarian groups. Nonetheless, they provided the blueprint for elitist schools in America.

Education and government were closely associated during the colonial era in American history. Here education was a powerful tool for social control. The Puritans dictated that their brand of Protestantism was funded by the government and that their religious tenths predominated. Accordingly, education within the New England colonial theocracy existed at three tiers: (1) elementary Bible schools, (2) classical Latin schools, and (3) colleges. The basic Bible school system was established under the Calvinist *Synod of Dort* doctrine (1618–1619). Under this resolution, Bible teaching was required for all children of White families with in-home instruction, as well as at church and in schools. Teachers were male but females were taught as well as males under this system.

The Massachusetts Bay Colony law of 1647 required towns to establish and support their own schools and to provide apprenticeship training and elementary Bible education for all free, White families. The law required towns comprised of 50 families or more to maintain an elementary school and for each town of 100 families to also provide a Latin preparatory school—the forerunner of contemporary high schools. These preparatory (prep) schools were feeder schools to Harvard College which was established in 1636. In 1650, the Connecticut Colony followed suit, and soon this system of public education became the standard in the New England colonies. These schools were for the established members of society, those recognized by the Congregationalist. The colleges produced the ministers and community leaders during this era of the State and Church theocracy that governed New England well beyond its colonial roots. The poor, on the other hand, were absorbed into society through apprenticeship training, a system based on the British 1562 Statutes of Artificers and the 1601 Poor Laws.[7]

It was the Quakers, however, who initiated the concept of universal education in the American colonies where it was first developed in the Middle Colonies (New York, New Jersey, and Pennsylvania) by the Society of Friends with the establishment of the William Penn Charter School in 1701 and the Trinity Church School in 1710. The Middle Colonies were more culturally and religiously diverse, hence the Dutch, French, Germans, Scandinavians, and non-Calvinist English brought a degree of tolerance not seen in the more homogeneous New England and Southern colonies. A number of colleges emerged in the Middle Colonies including the College of New Jersey (Princeton), King's College (Columbia), Queen's College (Rutgers), and the College of Philadelphia (University of Pennsylvania). In 1745, German Moravians established the first seminary for girls and, along with the Quakers, broke the mold of education being reserved solely for White, landed gentry males. The Quakers also provided educational opportunities for the children, both boys and girls, of former slaves.[8]

Education in the colonial South was primarily a private affair arranged by the plantation owners with the White elite providing tutors and special schooling for their children. The absence of a viable middle class restricted the development of public schools forcing poor Whites and Black slaves to rely on the charity, if any, of the plantation owners. Consequently, population of the Southern colonies was less educated than the other colonies. Even then, some Blacks were afforded limited access to education and apprenticeships laying the foundation for the emerging Black bourgeoisie. These efforts were initiated by the Society for the Propagation of the Gospel in Foreign Parts and similar religious-based organizations.[9] Given these marked differences, educational difference provided a major task for those establishing a new single federal system of government. This meant challenging the strong theocracies that existed throughout the former colonies, especially New England and the South, where religion provided the foundation for their respective society orders. Even then, the separation of church and state was a slow process with Protestantism emerging as the de facto Church of America.

The educational system based on the Protestant Ethic provided the basis for American socialization along with its system of stratification, status and role expectations. Thus, the race, sex, religious, and class format that emerged during the colonial era, later followed the U.S. Civil War and emancipation and the massive influx of non-Protestant emigrants in the late 19th and early 20th centuries. Basic literacy, based on the four "Rs"—reading, "riting" (writing), "rithmetic" (mathematics), religion (Bible for Protestants; Catechism for Catholics)—with its beginnings in the 1840s slowly spread across the nation while higher education began to expand during and immediately following the U.S. Civil War. The Morrill Act of 1862 established the state land grant university system addressing the need for scientific, agricultural, and industrial training through the sale of public land to be used for the creation of agricultural and mechanical colleges. The Second Morrill Act of 1890 extended the land grant provisions to the southern states. The establishment of state universities opened up higher education to working and middle-class people who would not otherwise be accepted to the "elite" Ivy League schools. The Morrill Act movement led to the establishment of three-year normal schools designed to prepare elementary and secondary teachers. The normal schools transitioned to four-year teachers' colleges during the 20th century. In 1876, Johns Hopkins was created as a graduate university establishing yet another trend.

The Second Morrill Act authorized the creation of Black universities resulting in 17 southern states developing separate Black agricultural and mechanical (engineering) A&M universities which joined the growing ranks of the "Historical Black Colleges and Universities" (HBCUs) which once numbered 121. The HBCUs not only provided the needed teachers, doctors, lawyers, and engineers during the post-Civil War Jim Crow era, they were the foundation of the Black bourgeois. A separate Catholic educational system also emerged in the United States before the Civil War with the advent of French-Canadians working in the New England mills and the survivors of the Irish Famine. Run by Priests, Brothers, and Nuns, these parochial schools were totally funded by the parishes with no state or federal funds. They provided bilingual instructions up to the sixth grade for the working classes but also provided eighth-grade and high school education for the middle classes. Catholic colleges and universities sprang up as well contributing to the Catholic bourgeois with nearly 200 schools comprising the "Association of Catholic Colleges and Universities" (ACCU). A few Jewish colleges and universities, like Brandeis in Massachusetts, were established to accommodate the influx of European immigrants in the late 1800s—early 1900s and following the World War II, but their numbers are small in comparison to "Protestant" and Catholic facilities of higher education. While the normal schools catered primarily to women, separate colleges and universities also grew in the post-Civil War era notably for White women notably in the East and South, while universities in Iowa, Maine, Michigan, Wisconsin, and Cornell in New York were early co-ed facilities. The GI Bill, created during the World War II, had an educational component that opened the doors of colleges and universities to millions of veterans who otherwise would not have had this opportunity.[10]

Even then, the elite still dominated the most desired schools gaining entrance through exclusive preparatory schools—the boarding schools. The main point here is that education per se is not secular regardless of however its presentation. In Canada, they have long made a distinction between "Protestant" and "Catholic" schools within its public school educational system. This recognizes the fact that sectarian ethno-methodologies use the educational system as the primary socialization mechanism for its members to "know their place" within the prevailing social order—both within the group and in relations to outside groups within their world order. Clearly, education promotes the social stratification hierarchy along with its prescriptions for sex, race/ethnic, class, and caste divisions. Regarding race, class, elitism, and privilege, boarding schools played a significant role at either end of the social spectrum. Boarding schools emerged as special institutions for both the elite and racial minorities. Boarding schools were used to perpetuate the power elite in America, on the one hand, and to forcefully resocialize former Black slaves and American Indians, on the other hand. Here, we compare and contrast two different boarding schools and their mandate. The Hampton/Carlisle in Virginia and St. Paul's School (SPS) in New Hampshire illustrate this process.

The Hampton/Carlisle Boarding School

In 1866, U.S. Civil War Brevet Brigadier General, Samuel Chapman Armstrong, was appointed as an agent of the Freedmen's Bureau whose role was to provide ways and methods for newly freed Blacks to function in society during the Reconstruction Era. General Armstrong was subsequently placed in charge of the Freedmen's camp at Hampton, Virginia. It was here that he established the

Hampton Normal and Industrial Institute in 1868 with a curriculum based on mental and manual training. A decade later, during the Indian Wars (1862–1892), the War Department began sending Indian youth to the Hampton Institute. The first Indians to arrive were 17 boys who were transferred from Fort Marion, a federal Indian prison located in St. Augustine, Florida. Captain Richard H. Pratt was the person responsible for this transfer.

When it was determined that the mix of Black Freedmen and incarcerated American Indians was not a good one, Pratt, with the blessings of General Armstrong, established a separate facility adjacent to the Hampton Institute solely for Indian students. General Armstrong acquired a 400-acre campus adjacent to the Hampton Institute for Pratt's Indian Institute, *Carlisle,* serving as the *Indian Branch* of the parent Hampton Institute. Carlisle began as a separate Indian boarding school in April 1878 with a contingent of Indian prisoners from the Kiowa, Comanche, Arapahoe, Caddo, and Cheyenne tribes. Later, Sioux prisoners from Pine Ridge (Ogallala) and Rosebud (Brule) tribes, in what is now South Dakota, joined student population. Soon a cross-representation of Indian youth arrived at the Carlisle Barracks in Pennsylvania including members of Geronimo's imprisoned band, the Chiricahua which arrived in 1887 at the conclusion of the Apache campaign.

Pratt's school at Carlisle clearly portrayed the rich history of this era and the long battle of the U.S. government attempting to resolve its *Indian Problem* plaguing it from the onset of the Republic. Major tribal leaders like Spotted Tail, Red Cloud, and Geronimo were against Indian boarding schools in general and Carlisle in particular viewing them as instruments designed at destroying Indian cultural and heritage—what would be currently knows as *cultural genocide.* Nonetheless, Carlisle came to epitomize the off-reservation, federally subsidized and religious controlled boarding schools of the time. During the 30-year Indian Wars, Indian policy was transferred from military (War Department) to civilian (Department of Interior) control, and by the 1880s, the number of federally supported Indian schools reached over 100, including a dozen boarding schools like Carlisle created from abandoned military facilities. Most notably of these facilities are Haskell Indian School located in Lawrence, Kansas, and the Moravian Mission School in Bethel, Alaska.[11]

Both the United States and Canada used the harsh boarding school system as a form of cultural genocide first, and as a tool for the enculturation of a racial caste system within their larger society secondly. This was not an attempt at integrating Indigenous peoples into White society. If this was the case, then they would have enfranchised American Indians giving them the same rights and privileges as Whites. Not so, given that American Indians were not federally enfranchised until 1924 while numerous states continued to keep them disenfranchised for 50 more years. This clearly was an effort to prohibit Indian youth from being socialized according to their respective tribal traditions, including language acquisition, rites, customs, and rituals. The process was to create psychological and cultural havoc while, at the same time, teaching Indians their place as "third-class" citizens vis-à-vis others, notably Whites, in American and Canadian society. This process departed markedly from the Jim Crow system applied to Blacks and Hispanics. While the Jim Crow system maintained the traditional caste and class differences through discriminatory "pig laws/Black Code" and grossly inadequate funding for Black as well as Hispanic schools, these schools, nonetheless, were taught by their own people who were able to retain a greater degree of their cultural heritage. This was not the case with American Indians who were not able to control their own schools until the mid-1970s under *Indian Self-Determination* at a time when the Boarding school experiment already nearly destroyed their cultural heritage.

While this plan succeeded to a great extent in destroying many tribal languages and traditions, it unexpectedly, and unintentionally, served to destroy long-held Euro-American tool of exploiting these intertribal factions in the conquest of tribes and the stealing of their lands and resources.

Hence, an unintended, latent function of forced boarding school incarceration led to the dissolution of these long-held intertribal factions by virtue of the mixing of children and youth from traditionally hostile tribes together; helping them to forge new friendships and relationships, including marriage. And by breaking down traditional intertribal barriers, these "incarcerated" Indians came to rely on the remnants of each other's surviving cultural attributes in forging a new survival network known as *Pan-Indianism*.[12]

Pan-Indianism began as a tool for collective survival among rival tribes being forced off their traditional lands by Whites. In the United States, this process can be traced to the 1830 Indian Removal Bill forcing eastern tribes to the collective dumping ground known as "Indian Territory" (later the state of Oklahoma). The larger south-eastern tribes, Cherokee, Creek, Choctaw, Chickasaw, and Seminole, were a diverse linguistic group that became known collectively as "The Five Civilized Tribes." This label was assigned to them given that they reluctantly adopted Euro-American ways in order to retain their traditional pre-Columbus lands. History tells us that this was not the case and White pressure to take their land and forcibly remove them become known as the "Trails of Tears." Once removed from President Jefferson's designated "Indian territory," these tribes began to share methods of adaptation to both their forced resocialization (civilization) and relocation. Further adaptations occurred during the U.S. Civil War which further devastated these tribes.[13]

While these earlier experiences contributed to the evolving Pan-Indian movement, none seemed sufficient, in themselves, to account for the transformation that occurred in the latter part of the 20th century. It took events like the boarding schools and the World War II to initiate the magnitude of the movement that truly transcended the historical tribal divisions that existed in the past. During the 1940s and 1950s, thousands of young Indian servicemen, many products of the boarding schools, returned to their reservations and homes with a different, more broader perspective on world events leading to the creation in 1944 of the National Congress of American Indians (NCAI). Although other White-sponsored Indian organizations preceded the NCAI, this was the first viable Indigenous-sponsored program. Later, in the 1960s, during the turbulent Civil Rights and Anti-War Movements, a more vocal, youth-oriented group emerged—the National Indian Youth Council (NIYC) along with its more radical arm—the American Indian Movement (AIM).

This radicalism led to the occupation of Alcatraz in the 1960s; the takeover of the Bureau of Indian Affairs (BIA) in Washington, DC, in 1972; and ill-fated ten-week siege of Wounded Knee on the Pine Ridge Sioux Reservation in South Dakota. Nonetheless, it took these actions to put an end to the Indian Boarding School program, a phenomenon articulated by the American Indian Historical Society:

> The only federally-controlled educational system in this nation is that directed by the Bureau of Indian Affairs, the so-called Indian schools, both boarding and day schools, from elementary to high school levels. The question as to how this fits into the democratic concept of education has been raised by the American Indian Historical Society already, and has been answered: It does not fit. Nevertheless, to change these schools, a proposal has been to put them under the direction of the tribal governing bodies and the Indian communities, under boards of education controlled by the people themselves. The situation at present in that the BIA controls the schools, the curriculum, the choice of textbooks, and the students themselves.[14]

The American Indian Historical Society played an important role and had influence that led to passage of the Indian Education Act in 1972 and the Indian Self-Determination and Education

Assistance Act in 1975 leading to local tribal control of Indian education and schools in Indian Country.[15]

SPS

The mid-19th century also saw the emergence of America's Aristocrats answer to the elite English Public School preparatory school system. This system was on a higher echelon than the Latin High Schools and Academies that were the feeder schools to colleges and universities at the time prior to the advent of high schools and compulsory education for everyone. Here, a distinction was made between educating the general populace via grammar/elementary schools and high schools in that the preparatory secondary schools promoted a classical curriculum that taught the linguistics of high-status professional status—that required for religious leaders, lawyers, and those of the medical profession. Latin, and related languages, provided the foundation for exclusivity in higher education comprising the argot of these elitist professions prior to mid-20th century and the rapid democratization of education via the GI Bill and similar resources. Accordingly, SPS was part of the select elitist prep schools today ranking among the top 10 of elite Ivy League feeder schools along with the currently top ranked Phillips Exeter Academy also in New Hampshire. While Phillips Exeter Academy traces its origin to 1781, SPS had its origins in 1856.

SPS began as an Episcopal School with a curriculum of Latin, Greek, and Mathematics. Its mandate was to instill the privilege status of the upper-class male in American society. In this sense, it was much like the Hampton/Carlisle Institutes in that its role was to reinforce the strict social strata at the time—"learning one's place in society." Sociologist and SPS alum and author of *Privilege: The Making of an Adolescent Elite at St. Paul's School,* Shamus Rahman Khan, explains this 19th century as follows:

> Boarding schools helped families construct and solidify ties with one another and ensure that their children were well equipped to participate in activities with other elites. They were protectionist institutions aimed at providing not only the knowledge required to be successful but the culture, morality, and social ties that were essential to the American elite. The fact that the mere accumulation of capital was not the overwhelming interest of this old American elite is also a nod to an older, more aristocratic version of an elite who seeks to create barriers that prevent others from joining their rolls.[16]

SPS, with its 2,000-acre rural setting a few miles from the New Hampshire capital, Concord, was established in New Hampshire during Franklin Pierce's presidency, and it reflected Pierce's Southern leanings supportive of slavery as the status quo. These conservative sentiments were articulated by August Heckscher, an alum and official historian of the school, who describes SPS' original epistemology as departing from the English elite public schools at the time in that SPS was more austere and authoritarian. This perspective reflected the tenths of Protestant predestination at the time which provided the basis for class and caste structure in America. This was reflected in the philosophy and practices of its first Rector, the Reverend Henry Coit, during his 39-year tenure, a worldview shared by his contemporaries running the Black and Indian boarding schools at Hampton and Carlisle. Austerity, authoritarianism, and charity were combined within a classical curriculum that prepared the White elite males in their future roles in life. While struggling through its own difficult economic straits, Rector Coit was instrumental in providing for the orphaned children of fathers killed or missing during the U.S. Civil War. Working in concert with the city of Concord, SPS provided a home for these children in April 1866—the Concord

Orphanage—"Coit House." In 1874, the home was transferred to a board of trustees under the Episcopal Diocese.[17]

SPS continued to grow in both stature and wealth through the trials and tribulations of two World Wars often recruiting faculty ("Masters") and even Rectors from its best students thereby continuing to insulate itself from outside influences that may pose a threat to their preparatory perspective. This shield of protection along with its religious orthodoxy ended during the turbulent civil rights and anti-war era of the 1960s and 1970s. The stage for change was actually set in 1956 when SPS hired the Reverend John Walker of Detroit as its first Black faculty (Master). He served in this capacity until 1966. The first Black student was admitted to SPS two years following Walker's hire. The Reverend Walker left SPS to become Canon of the National Cathedral in Washington, DC, and, later, Bishop of Washington, DC. In 1972, he became the first Black SPS Trustee.[18]

The turmoil of the 1960s and 1970s penetrated the once seemingly impregnable shroud engulfing SPS especially reactions to the assassinations of President J.F. Kennedy, his brother Robert, and Martin Luther King, Jr. Like their counterparts elsewhere, SPS student and faculty began pushing for change while student lifestyles changed as well, including drug experimentation:

> By the mid-1960s something like a revolutionary mood was developing in Millville (SPS) ... a handful of activists, influenced by politically conscious, younger members of the faculty, voiced the mounting mood of dissent. Finally, several strongly individualistic sixth form presidents were endeavouring to bring St. Paul's into line with what was going on at other schools and colleges. The school administration responded to the growing dissidence, not by searching for culprits but by pushing forward with changes that had been in progress for several years. These included freely granted weekends away from school, as well as experiments in reducing the number of compulsory chapel services. Requirements for seated meals, enforced study hours and formal rules of dress were also relaxed. At the same time efforts were made to increase the number of minority students and—not lease—to bring in groups of girl students during the winter term.[19]

These times witnessed a transformation at SPS including a secularization of its strict religious schedule, an increased minority student population, and being one of the first of the elite boarding schools to go co-ed. Much of the success of this transition is credited to its new Rector, William ("Wild Bill") Oates, who was selected from the teaching ranks. A Harvard graduate but not an ordained minister, Oates helped smooth out the path to a more contemporary secular curriculum and the admission of the first 19 female students in January 1971 which included two Black students. The increasingly growing minority students, mostly Black males, choose to reside in their own dorm so as to better maintain their ethnic culture. Oates was able to suppress efforts by students to radically change SPS traditions. As a compromise, the dress code was relaxed, and the number of "seated meals" and "compulsory chapels" was reduced, and a black history course was added to the curriculum.

In 1982, during the Reagan years, SPS' ninth Rector swung to schools to its more conservative origins with the selection of Charles H. ("Kelley aka Chuck") Clark former Dean of the Berkeley Divinity School at Yale. With his selection came a reawakening of the school's Episcopal tradition. Clearly, this effort to eradicate the changes made under the Oates administration under Clark's authoritarian regime, including increased security, a watchtower, guards, and high-power sweep-lights did little to diminish the student subculture of challenging these stricter rules as Heckscher noted:

> All this was in the background of a landscape otherwise sunny and placid: too sunny to please some of the more cynical, "St. Paul's School has a very intricate camouflage system," a student explained in the *Pelican*. "The school hides problems from the outside world, and we hide problems from the teachers, each other, and ourselves."[20]

A unique feature of SPS is its Advanced Studies Program (ASP) initiated in 1957 during the Sputnik scare of the Cold War. This program provides an opportunity for gifted New Hampshire high school students to attend a specialized summer school at a reasonable cost (with a liberal financial aid program) in a concentrated area of their interest. This program is for students who have completed their junior year allowing them to seek out quality colleges and universities once they graduate. The ASP graduates are often recruited by these schools given them an advantage that their elite counterparts at SPS have. It is a great opportunity for working and middle-class families to gain access to a quality education for their children. The ASP had 242 students from 72 high schools in 2019. The program went online in 2020 due to the COVID-19 pandemic with 120 students from 51 high schools. Generally, the gender distribution is 60% female and 40% male students.

The Mechanism of Privilege and Entitlement

Audiences and Circles of Influence

It is generally accepted that our "existence" is determined by how we are defined within our social subset which determines our social status and corresponding role expectations. Here, the core factor of our existential persona is *purpose*—who are we and what is expected of us. To this end, we rely on audience feedback for our identity. Our audiences, on the other hand, involve concentric levels of influence—from intimate to generalized. George Herbert Mead, a 20th-century American sociologist, articulated a theory of human development and our respective levels of audiences. His theory of development corresponded loosely with that of Sigmund Freud whereby as infants we are genetically wired to be dependent and demanding. This is the "I" and it corresponds with Freud's "Id." Next, as we develop as children, our audience of influence is expanded beyond the family to that of school-age peers, teachers, and the like. Mead termed this stage as the "Me" where we learn the basic mechanisms for appropriate socialization as prescribed by our primary groups. In Freud's schematic, this is when the "ego" begins to develop. In Mead's last stage, the "Self" emerges having now inculcated the norms and role expectations of our primary and secondary audiences. To Freud, this is our "Superego."[21]

The Austrian/German "Gestalt School" (ax Wertheimer, Kurt Koffka, Wofgang Kohler, Kurt Levin) linked our existence beyond pure existentialism linking it with relevant phenomenon within our spheres of socialization. The Gestalt School based their "field theory," "insights," and "Phi Phenomenon" on the physical sciences. In a nut shell, they articulated the significance of the influence of others within our social orbit noting that the group was greater than the sum of its individual components. These psychologists linked existentialism with phenomenology through their concept of the "feedback loop" whereby the individual gains insights into themselves via audience responses to their behavior and performance. Accordingly, we derive feedback from the different audiences that influence our behavior. The first and most intimate level are the expectations from our significant others like our family followed by the expectations of our peers. Beyond that are what is termed "generalized others" which connotes our perception of a larger audience within society and even beyond.[22]

Added to this conceptual scheme is the works of Ralph Linton who articulated the terms "status" and "role." Here, Linton noted that the functioning of societies is dependent on the presence of patterns of reciprocal relations between the individuals or groups of individuals. Behavioral expectations (role) are defined by the group in terms of status. Generally speaking, society defines two types of status—ascribed status versus achieved status. The former reflects our inherited, biological status such as age, height, race, ethnicity, gender, caste, class, etc. while the latter refers to our achievements as outlined by the group such as social strata, marital status, professional/occupational status, socioeconomic status, and the like. Roles represent the dynamic aspect of a status along with rights, duties, and expectations. In this sense, class, caste, privilege, and entitlements are elements of our status. Herbert Hyman noted that our behavioral expectations are usually driven by the group with which we psychologically identify our "reference group." However, this perceived status may differ from that assigned to us by the group from which we originated, sometimes making us an outcast from our group. Options for these individuals who feel excluded from their group include leaving their group of orientation and drifting to a more tolerant group. Durkheim noted that situations where a person feels totally isolated or alienated from their group often lead to a serious detachment of normlessness (anomie) which in its extreme results in suicide. Robert K. Merton addressed the issues associated with social structure and anomie in an article published in 1938 that addressed the concept of "relative deprivation," the process whereby we compare our status to those who hold similar status and the psychological anguish and, sometimes, trauma arising from this situation. Samuel Stouffer, in turn, led a massive social psychological study on American GIs during World War II and the role relative deprivation played in the mental stability of service personnel during and following this conflict.[23]

Social Structure and Institutional and Systemic Biases

Given that the family is the primary agent of socialization, it provides us with the biases that we inherit from this powerful, subtle orientation to life, notably our epigenetic biases—those biases that are mainly autonomic not surfacing until an emotional crisis triggers their arousal. These values and biases, imbued by our mother's milk, provide the lens from which we perceive our personal reality, in essence, our persona—our existence. These are the emotional signals emitted from our primitive brain, the limbic system, that influence our cerebral thinking processes. Max Weber alluded to this process when addressing the influences of our "family of orientation" stating that the existence of these biases obviates our being "value free" in our judgments. Hence, this subconscious process fuels our perception of reality and situations providing the foundation for our "Attribution Biases." Accordingly, our social experiences teach us "our place" in society as well as teaching us the rules relevant to achieving social status, a process involving inculcating the dynamics of inclusion/exclusion, social mobility, achieved and ascribed status, and, where relevant, caste and class.[24]

Generally speaking, primitive societies, historical and contemporary, based status within a clan or extended family setting. Once villages, towns, and cities emerged, secondary institutions came into play with their own status and role expectations, including privilege and entitlements. In this scenario, behavioral expectations take on the element of ethical standards and trust associated with various roles. Bankers, doctors, lawyers, educators, law enforcement, judges, military personnel, etc. are held to a certain level of professional standards by the members of society they serve. Yet these institutions do not exist in a vacuum. Status takes on another element of competition within each organization and even between organizations. Not to be ignored is the influence of holding an "affiliate" status such as being associated or married to someone of higher status such as the nurse marring the successful doctor. Organizations often create elaborate hierarchies of "esoteric" status and even "enhanced" status. Status stratification enhances the relative standing of both the organization and its members; hence, the efforts made to protect these institutions at any cost, including fostering a culture of silence, secrecy, and concealment. Any attack on the organization is seen as a personal assault by its constituency, thus fostering a sort of in-group entrenchment against outside criticism following Simmel's theorem that out-group hostility increases in-group cohesion. Here, any sign of a threat sees the organization closing rank, strongly discouraging any dissent, and disparaging and punishing whistleblowers, along with efforts to cover up alleged misdoings.

This phenomenon pertains to academia, law enforcement agencies, religious organizations, even the Boy Scouts of America. The protection of ethical miscreants, even when they are few, is seen as paramount to the preservation of the special status and privileges afforded the institution by society in general. Within institutions, status enhancement is often used to promote one's professional status to the general public as well. A prime example is the recent phenomenon of ranking police officials, regardless of how small the force, and Sheriffs, donning the stars of high-ranking military officers, even five-stars, thereby greatly enhancing the perception of both their status and authority in addition to contributing to the militarization of law enforcement.[25] Esoteric status, in turn, pertains to the internal strata within organizations and professions. In academia, the strata include instructor, assistant, associate, and full professor status, along with emeritus and distinguished labels for productive careers within the tenured ranks. Nontenure track educators are generally listed as adjunct, clinical, affiliate, or visiting faculty. Other organization have similar administrative hierarchies with subordinate titles such as "assistant," "associate," "deputy," "senior," or "vice" as well as numerical designations such as "First Vice President" or a combination of these labels—"Associate Deputy Director." Correspondingly, agencies, institutional, and organizations have diluted standards contributing to inflated status among their ranks. Professions where once a master's degree sufficed as a "terminal degree" for public practice, like audiology and physical therapists, have now been elevated to the doctoral level and offered at academic institutions that would not otherwise qualify for doctoral level studies due to a lack of research and library resources, among other considerations. These additions to the doctoral ranks include those from the medical/clinical profession (Doctor of Osteopathic Medicine—D.O.s vs. M.D.s) and Psy.D. for professional psychologists who have not undergone the rigors of a Ph.D. program. Education also followed suit adding "easy" masters and doctorate programs so as to elevate the status of teachers and administrators, among others, offering the one-year Masters of Arts in Teaching (MAT). The MAT evolved as the answer to state boards of education requiring a master's for certification or licensure. It became a post-baccalaureate degree earned within a year and without a required thesis. This soon became the "terminal" degree for those in other academic disciplines who could not meet the demands for discipline-specific M.A. or M.S. degrees. The Doctor of Education (Ed.D.), Doctor of Arts (D.A.) and Doctor of Public Administration (D.P.A.) degrees followed this trend with these degrees offered mainly at colleges that otherwise do not qualify to offer Ph.D. degrees in addition to major state universities in their quest of getting a share on the lucrative "vanity degree" market.

The legal profession illustrates America's initiative in enhancing both the professional and academic of attorneys attending U.S. law programs. In the late 1960s, a major transformation occurred within the legal profession, notably the traditional bachelor of law degree, the L.L.B. (*Legum Baccalaureas*), was elevated to doctoral status with the creation of the J.D. (*Jurum Doctor*) despite the fact that the L.L.M. (*Legum Magister—Masters of Laws*) and L.L.D. (*Legum Doctor—Doctor of Laws*) remain the advanced law degrees. In the United States, the J.D. has competed with legitimate doctoral degrees within academia, notably in criminal justice and political sciences programs, even though it is viewed as either an advanced bachelor or as a master's degree in other countries recognizing the J.D. degree where it certainly is not held as the equivalent of earned research doctoral degrees or the L.L.M. or L.L.D. degrees. In the United States, some law schools now offer accelerated two-year J.D. degrees placing them on par with academic master's degree programs. Nonetheless, those with the J.D. degree as their "terminal" or highest degree wear the same three-chevron gown at graduations and formal functions, including Judges, as that of their real doctorate counterparts. Added to this phenomenon is the proliferation of unaccredited diploma mills that basically sell college degrees, including academic doctoral degrees. Another gimmick are professional mutual admiration societies that endorse each other for esoteric titles such as "best lawyer in America" awards which are then used as a marketing device when published in glossy magazines like *New Hampshire Magazine*—an offprint of Yankee Publishing. In this issue, hundreds of attorneys were listed as award winners.[26]

"Club Ed" and the Spoils of the Privileged Elite

Education and social status are closely correlated within developed nations including the United States. Educational status in Europe, for example, has long been the mechanism for setting class lines. A similar process existed in the American colonies with access to higher education available primarily for the members of the new American Aristocracy. Following independence, class and caste remained part and parcel of U.S. cultures and educational accessibility—the main tool for status discrimination. Today, with the democratization of higher education, professional status is available to those who can afford it. Even then, the power elites in American society continue to dominate the ranks of prestigious schools (prep schools, college, universities) creating a type of privilege entitlement allowing them to remain at the helm of the capitalist/political power structure. The *Legacy* admission process allows entry to even those who have marginal abilities creating a form of affirmative action for the rich and famous. The education of former U.S. President, George H. Bush (2001–2009) illustrates this phenomenon. It could be argued that his admission to Phillips Andover Academy, Yale, and Harvard Universities probably had more to do with his family's wealth and status than it did with academic merit.

Academic status is denoted by the addition of presumably earned degrees to the names of those holding these distinctions—M.D., J.D., Ph.D., Ed.D., etc. These labels are paramount to one's status in much of the world. In Europe, for example, those with both research doctorates and professorial rank generally have added both as prefaces to their title—"Doctor Professor French." With the proliferation of lesser doctorates in the United States, some with higher status doctorates (Ivy Leaguers and the like) deliberately omit their academic credential in a form of reverse elitist snobbery indicating that the general public remains beyond their preferred audience. This movement of esoteric status follows that of inclusive clubs like the Masons, Knights of Columbus, Elks, and Moose organizations where their rites and customs remain secret and meaningful only to its select audience. Ivy League elitism is seen as a reaction to degrees conferred by what they perceive as being "inferior" institutions, including State Universities, many of which have excellent facilities and faculty. Added to this mix, however, are the so-called Mickey Mouse leadership programs, some offered within education and criminal justice disciplines at these otherwise outstanding public institutions, including ranking flagship institutions.

William Henry Cosby, aka Bill Cosby, offers a prime example of these "lesser degrees" offered by an otherwise ranking flagship institution of higher education—the University of Massachusetts at Amherst. The standard for the move from quantitative research-based doctorates to the "create your own degree" vanity Ed.D. doctorate market was adopted by the University of Massachusetts in the 1970s. According to his biography, Cosby was born in Germantown, Pennsylvania, on July 12, 1937. He left school in the 10th grade to join the U.S. Navy where he completed his high school degree via a corresponding course. Once released from active duty, Cosby earned his undergraduate at Temple University under a football scholarship. He went on to earn his Masters of Education degree at the University of Massachusetts–Amherst. Cosby's 1976 Ed.D. dissertation was titled: *An Integration of the visual media via "Fat Albert and the Cosby Kids" into the elementary school curriculum as a teaching aid and vehicle to achieve increased learning.* The 267-page dissertation had a text of 148 pages, a bibliography containing 71 items, and a 117 supplementary portfolio. His research consisted of a questionnaire sent out to 122 teachers and 19 others. The questionnaire was designed to determine the effectiveness of the Fat Albert scripts as a curriculum tool in elementary school classrooms. While the questionnaire lent itself to tests of significance analysis (Likert-type scales; chi square, etc.)—none were conducted. Instead percentages were used with no tests of significant differences determined. Moreover, no research design was present and no in-group or within-group analysis indicted. Nonetheless, this model soon became the norm for similar Ed.D. programs within education.[27]

Eventually, more colleges and universities began offering these diluted Ed.D. degrees mainly in the area of education administration for primary and secondary principals and public school superintendents. During the 1990s, this market grew so great that the title was changed to "Educational Leadership" and began to be offered at numerous colleges and universities that were otherwise only certified to teach primarily undergraduate and a scattering of master's degrees, mostly in education. In North Carolina with its university chartered in 1789 and now consisting of a 16-campus system statewide has made the Ed.D. available at some its non-doctoral conferring "four-year" schools like Western Carolina University. These leadership doctorates also depart from the individualized research doctorates in that they are group endeavors comprised of a cohort of peers pursuing the Ed.D. together. The general admission requirements for these cohort "Leadership" programs are the same as those for master's degree programs with the prerequisite of a master's degree in school administration, supervision, or curriculum. These programs often allow for a portfolio in lieu of any meaningful thesis or dissertation. It appears that these programs are designed to inflate the status of school administrators and do little to reflect on true academic or intellectual qualifications as a 1998 *U.S. News & World Report* attests:

> Our schools of education have been a national scandal for many years, but it's odd that they are rarely front-and-center in our endless debate about failing schools. The right talks about striving and standards, the left talks about equal funding and classroom size, but few talk much about the breeding grounds for school failure—the trendy, anti-achievement, oppression-obsessed, feel-good, esteem-ridden, content-free schools of education.[28]

The quest for educational status in order to enhance one's social, political, or job status went beyond the teaching profession and soon was seen as the road to promotion in such diverse occupations and professions as law enforcement, the military, and other aspect of public service and private enterprise. This demand led to the proliferation of "diploma mills," many of dubious standards. John Bear, a leading authority on alternative college degrees, noted that there are more than 300 unaccredited so-called academic institutions operating in the United States, some offering online courses and degrees, while many are fake diploma mills selling degrees for thousands of dollars. Even state government consortiums and the U.S. Military have bought into the online education scheme. Western Governor University (WGU) is an unaccredited internet school offering master's degree programs in education. Started in 1998, WGU has the backing of the governors of 13 states offering degrees to anyone who passes its tests. In 2000, the U.S. Army established the Army University Online competing with the already successful United States Armed Forces Institute (USAFI) that offers courses and degrees sponsored by the University of Maryland and Wisconsin. Even the U.S. Marine Corps now has its own Marine Corps University offering master's degrees to field-grade officers.

Bear lists the top fake schools in the United States such as Bernadean University, the University of San Gabriel Valley, Southland University, LaSalle University, Edison University, Open University of America, Hamilton University, Columbia Pacific University, Concord University of Law, Cardean University, Trinity College and University, and Columbia State University. He noted that fake schools usually establish mail drops in states that do not stringently regulate schools of higher education. California, Hawaii, Louisiana, and Wyoming are prime targets for these fake schools. Clearly, this is an international problem plaguing many nations. Part of the problem is that these fake schools are not vetted properly when marketed in prominent periodicals such as *Business Week*, *Economist*, *Time*, *Forbes*, *Newsweek*, *Money*, *Investor's Business Daily*, and *USA Today*. Adding to this problem, phony replacement degrees listing prominent colleges and universities are available via the mail from these bogus sites. Diploma mills often find loopholes regarding accreditation listing accrediting agencies not regulated by the U.S. Department of Education such as the International Accreditation Agency (IAC), the American Council of Private Colleges and Universities, the Association for Online Academic Excellence, the World Council of Global Education, and World Association of Universities and Colleges. Among this group were religious schools of dubious accreditation and quality, known as *Christian Degree Mills.* Perhaps the most notorious diploma mill was the now defunct *Trump University.* The problem of enhanced or outright bogus degrees is not unique to the United States. Prior to the breakup of the Soviet Union and the former Yugoslavia, little was known about the quality or validity of academic and professional degrees from these entities leading to the 1999 Bologna Accord, as part of the Lisbon Recognition Convention, whereby[29] European Council members established a standard for degree recognition especially within higher education. Those member states could now better evaluate the degrees stemming from the new states joining the European community. This was critical for those seeking advanced degrees or employment outside of the former Soviet or Yugoslav states.[29]

Status and Role Exploitation

The holder of high status has a corresponding ethical responsibility to adhere to the standards of behavior associated with this privilege. Ethical breeches often stem from the exploitation of the perceived entitlements associated with this privilege leading to a breach of trust. Self-aggrandizement often comes into play here as members of the cohort vie for recognition within their organizational structure, a phenomenon common to political, academic, legal, business, and military entities. Competition being a strong element of human nature, people compare their relative status to that holding similar status fueling both in-group and out-group angst—aka "relative deprivation"—leading to vast market, both legitimate and bogus, to accommodate this need for peer acknowledgment. In academia, it is known as "publish or perish."

"Padding" one's curriculum vitae is a major problem. This is most common with administrative heads or grant directors who include their name on all, or most, of the articles produced by their department or agency, often disproportionately in relations to their personnel contribution to the research itself. The American Psychological Association (APA) called this practice out as plagiarism:

> 8.12 Publication Credit
>
> (a) Psychologists take responsibility and credit, including authorship credit, only for work they have actually performed or to which they have substantially contributed. (See also Standard 8.12b, Publication Credit.)
>
> (b) Principal authorship and other publication credits accurately reflect the relative scientific or professional contributions of the individuals involved, regardless of their relative status. Mere possession of an institutional position, such as department chair, does not justify authorship credit. Minor contributions to the research or to the writing for publications are acknowledged appropriately, such as in footnotes or in an introductory statement.
>
> (c) Except under exceptional circumstances, a student is listed as principal author on any multiple-authored article that is substantially based on the student's doctoral dissertation. Faculty advisors discuss publication credit with students as early as feasible and throughout the research and publication process as appropriate. (See also Standard 8.12b, Publication Credit.)
>
> 8.13 Duplicate Publication of Data
>
> Psychologists do not publish, as original data, data that have been previously published. This does not preclude republishing data when they are accompanied by proper acknowledgment.[30]

I was aware of this practice in my teaching, research, and practice experiences. While working as a staff psychologist in the New Hampshire neuropsychiatric units, it was dictated that all publications or research results were to be censored by administrative figures with their names added if resulting in publications. As an example, I wanted to replicate a study I did with Apache and Mexican-born elderly in the psychiatric unit of a nursing home in Arizona where I served as clinical director. My colleague, Robert Williams, a staff psychologist at the New Hampshire (psychiatric/neurological) Hospital, and I decided to apply this research to elderly dementia patients of French-Canadian descent, whose first language was French. In order to get permission to conduct the study, Dr. Williams had to include his Dartmouth-affiliated psychiatric supervisor, Dr. Richard Ferrell, as a co-author although he had no other role in the project than allowing us access to the subjects. Apparently, this is a standard practice for psychiatrists who also hold faculty status at Dartmouth Medical School/Dartmouth College.[31]

In my academic career, I found these constraints and demands to be more common within criminology/criminal justice settings than in either sociology or psychology. I was able to expose this practice during my tenure at Western New Mexico University when asked to provide a blind review on *Gangs: A Criminal Justice Approach*, a special work sponsored by the Academy of Criminal Justice Sciences published by Anderson Monography Series. The book editors were under the impression that all the contributions represented the original work of the submitting authors. However, in my review of the material it became clear that the authors, Chair and senior faculty member at New Mexico State University's criminal justice department, were not the original authors but rather that of graduate students. My review of the monograph appeared in the journal, *Criminal Justice Review*:

> My greatest disappointment, however, was with the Winfree and Mays selection. Despite the editors' call for original works, it appears that this selection on family and peer influences on gang involvement is merely a reanalysis of old data resulting from two 1992 master's theses produced by the authors' former students—and Winfree and Mays' footnote acknowledging

> the students in the "collection efforts during the data entry phase" falls far short of current ethnical expectations. A good guide on this matter is the APA's 1992 *Ethical Principles of Psychologists and Code of Conduct* … Hopefully there is a general consensus within criminal justice that these are obvious ethical considerations that we would like to see followed, especially in publications reflective of the ACJS.[32]

Apparently, the message has not gotten through to criminology and criminal justice faculty. In a recent journal article (Fall 2019) Tom Bartlett of *The Chronicle of Higher Education* called a Florida State University (FSU) faculty for "cooking the books" regarding the manipulation of data analysis in recent publications in the American Society of Criminology's (ASC) main publication—*Criminology*. "Cooking the books" refers to voodoo statistical manipulation but also the fact that this faculty seems to have his name on numerous other articles drawing attention to the issue stated above concerning proportionate responsibility for publications. The in-group club nature of these professional organizations, regardless of academic discipline, lends itself to the "circulation of the elite" among their self-ordained member cohort whereby a select few arrear disproportionately in their major publications. The Bartlett article also addresses the issue of the esoteric quasi-scientific research methods as a prerequisite for publications in these journals. There seems to be a trend for social science disciplines to overemphasize their "scientific rigor" via statistics in order to place themselves on an even keel with the physical sciences. Dealing with secondary analysis of massive data sets without the possibility of source verification coupled with measurements of attitudes and similar "soft" variables, social sciences deal primarily with nonparametric data, while their physical science counterparts deal with parametric data sets. While there are good nonparametric measures for normative and ranked data, there has been a movement, since the computerization of statistical packets, to apply parametric measures to nonparametric data sets treating normative data as if they are either zero based or having gone through the rigor for determining a variance of standard deviation.[33]

Privilege, Entitlement, and "Sexploitation"

The concept of male sexual privilege is rooted in past examples of *Droit du Seigneur* (Lord's right), aka *jus primae noctis* (right of the first night), where a high-ranking official, like the Lord of the Manor, had the right to have sexual intercourse with young women within his realm who were to leave his domain usually through marriage. Although eventually outlawed by the Roman Catholic Church, this practice continued among European colonists, including in the New World through the sexploitation of both American Indian and African slaves, including notables such as Thomas Jefferson. Indeed, Andres Resendez notes that the practice among the Spanish of capturing and enslaving Indian women, notably Apache, from the Southwest and northern Mexico, and force marching them in chain gangs (colleras) for the sex and domestic workers markets in more densely populated areas of Mexico and the Caribbean, unwittingly fueled the spread of epidemics in North America including the worst smallpox epidemic of 1775 to 1782 that devastated tribal groups and colonial settlements, including African slaves, from southern Mexico to Canada. Despite Mexico abolishing slavery in 1829 with the United States following suit in 1865, de facto sexual slavery of Indian and Black women continued unabated throughout the 19th century contributing to the chaos and family violence among segments of these populations.[34]

It appears that elements of the "Lord's right" have survived through the years to the present not only among White elites but elites throughout the world. An area of concern in the United States is the sexploitation of military personnel by their superiors. The closed society of the military where "rank has its privileges" coupled with the recent expansion of females into the military branches has greatly exasperated this problem. In the past, this was a hidden secret among male service personnel, just like it is in male prison settings, where the abused is often more fearful of the stigma of victimization than the psychological trauma from the abuse itself. This changed during the Gulf War era when the United States, in its all-volunteer military, witnessed its largest deployment of women, many sent to combat zones. The Second Gulf War witnessed the largest deployment of women to combat zones with many serving as part of a federalized National Guard unit in Iraq or Afghanistan. Female service personnel serving in the 1990s to the present changed forever the subservient nurse image distinguishing themselves in air combat. In 2005, Sergeant Leigh Ann Hester became the first woman to receive the Silver Star decoration (the third highest decoration for Valor) since World War II cited for killing three enemy combatants in an attack on her support unit in Iraq. The Gulf Wars also witnessed the lifting of rank restrictions resulting in female generals and admirals with Major General Maggie Woodward being the first woman to command a combat air operation in 2011 in Operation Odyssey Dawn—the coalition force attack on Colonel Gaddafi 's forces during the Libyan civil war.[35]

Sexual abuse has been an unfortunate consequence of both domestic and foreign military deployments. In foreign deployments, including combat zones, prostitution fills part of this need. This was a dimension of the Gulf Wars with the increased numbers of female Guard personnel being the bait for sexual abuse by their male counterparts, including superiors. The military culture fosters a rape-prone environment within the military caste system. A 2010 Department of Defense (DoD) report indicated an 11% increase in reported sexual assault in the military that year with a 16% increase among those U.S. troops serving in Iraq and Afghanistan. The problem was so pervasive that the Care for Victims of Sexual Assault Task Force was established by the DoD in 2004 resulting in the creation of the Sexual Assault Response and Prevention Office (SAPRO) with the mandate of providing training and educational programs, treatment and support systems for victims, and establishing system accountability.

A major failing of these efforts to date has been the male chain of command and its inherent bias against female service personnel. Nonetheless, efforts are being made by the Veterans Administration (VA) to address this issue. Since 2008, the VA has been in the forefront of treatment for Military Sexual Trauma (MST). It is now recognized that the trauma associated with MST goes beyond rape and sexual assault to include unwanted sexual touching or grabbing, threatening offensive remarks about a person's body (body shaming), or other sexual activities such as threatening. The VA recognizes that MST is a form of post-traumatic stress disorder (PTSD) and can affect a person's mental and physical health for many years if not addressed properly. The VA provides free, confidential counseling and treatment to both male and female veterans for mental health and physical conditions related to experience of MST.[36]

Sexploitation in Academia

The systematic exploitation of female students, staff, and faculty has a long history in academia in America and beyond. A classic example is not giving adequate credit for research and publications by male colleagues. But a more significant problem is the view that male faculty are entitled to seduce females within their orbit of influence—a sort of privilege that appears to be pervasive within the realm of academia. A popular justification is that girls ask for sexual attention by virtue of their dress and appearance. Granted, the co-ed campus culture is sexually charged due mainly to the age and hormones of students of all genders, but it is foolhardy to place the blame specifically on co-eds. Another factor in faculty/student relations, albeit rare, can be explained by the clinical process known as *transference*—the unconscious assignment of others of feelings that were originally associated with important figures such as parents, etc. This would explain student attention toward faculty. *Countertransference* is the clinical process whereby the therapist, or faculty, attaches their unconscious feelings and needs to the client, or student. Regardless of the mechanism of action, sexual abuse within academia is known and shared within this particular environment regardless if you subscribe to these subcultural rituals or not.[37]

My awareness of this phenomenon occurred during my graduate studies in sociology where the sexual exploits of noted sociologists like C. Wright Mills and W.I. Thomas were spoken of as a "badge of honor." C. Wright Mills died in 1962; three years prior to my entry into college following my Marine Corps service so his sexual exploits were still fresh subcultural fodder. He was attributed to having sex with female students at night on his office desk at Columbia University with the lights on providing a show for his outside audience thus adding to his macho status. W.I. Thomas, who died in 1947, was part of the famous Chicago School of Social Psychology. His image gained notoriety within sociological circles surrounding rumors of his contacting a venereal disease while observing second-generation "unadjusted" girls within the various ethnic enclaves in the Chicago area. True or not these macho images seem to have only enhanced their professional images while also verifying the norms of privilege entitlement for aspiring male academics.[38]

The sexploitation of female students is also a common practice, within other academic environments, notably where corruption is institutionalized. One region for these abuses is Southern and Eastern Europe which I observed during two Fulbright experiences and conferences. While the Bologna Accord strives to address bogus and otherwise questionable academic credential in these emerging democracies in the 1990s, it did not provide sufficient filters that could detect sexploitation of female students by male faculty. The European system differs from that of the United States in that what the United States terms "colleges"—those disciplines that comprise a university—are called "faculties" within academic units in Europe. Faculty heads, aka, Deans, hold considerable control over their domain and often are political appointments. Another departure from the American academic system is that student grades are not submitted directly to a university registrar but rather are held by the student in their "Index (Indeks) book" which they present personally to their professor for his/her to sign, thereby verifying their attendance and grade for that particular course. It is within this process that the potential for faculty "sextortion" prevails. Here, grades, or grade adjustments, are contingent upon either monetary extortion (mainly for male students) or sex (mainly for female students). While this practice exists, it is unfair to assume that it is widespread among all faculty. Nonetheless, the fact remains that this practice is *known* by other faculty, if not, most of the faculty. And by silently condoning it allows it to continue unabated. This reflects the nature of "institutionalized audience effect" where in-group members are reluctant to publically expose "bad members" since they fear this would taint the entire faculty. By the same token, administrators at all levels also apply pressure to keep these events under wrap, again to protect the institutions and their reputation. Any sign of a threat, the organization closes rank and discourages dissent with threats of exclusion from the group. These actions are counter to the responsibility and trust associated with the privilege status associated with these positions and therefore represent grossly unethical behaviors. Despite these ethical responsibilities, it must be recognized that sexual exploitation is a strong human emotion representing a group dynamic that is likely to continue to occur in agencies and institutions that do not provide adequate oversight and an objective outside ethicists to monitor their operations. This includes prep schools, colleges, and universities in the United States.

The previously mentioned *#Me Too movement* set the stage for the disclosure of these abuses, some that have simmered for years at prominent academic institutions including the University of California–Irvine (UC-Irvine), Michigan State University (MSU), and Dartmouth College. Once exposed action usually followed such as that at UC-Irvine with the removal of faculty and administrators accused of sexual misconduct. It was the allegations leveled against Larry Nassar, the U.S. Gymnastics doctor at MSU, that drew the most attention to the problem of sexploitation within academia, its prevalence and attempts to cover up. The notoriety surrounding the MSU sexual abuse allegations was that the program attracted youth, including children, to the highly regarded U.S. Gymnastics program, including many from outside the college student population. Since Nassar's exposure in 2016 over 150 women have come forward with accusations of sexual abuse by Dr. Nassar which resulted in his conviction to a lengthy sentence tantamount to life imprisonment. The cover-up by MSU administrators included the then president, Lou Anna K. Simon. Simon was forced to resign in the wake of the scandal and was later charged with felony and misdemeanor counts for her role in the scandal only to have these charges dismissed by an Eaton County judge. Nassar's immediate supervisor, Dr. William Strapel, also implicated in the sex abuse of girls, was convicted of a felony and misdemeanor charges but ultimately ended up serving less than eight months of his sentence before being released.[39]

Dartmouth College Psychologists

Dartmouth College long had a "party school" reputation—one portrayed in the 1978 *National Lampoon's Animal House* which propelled actor John Belushi to fame. Drinking, wild partying, and sex became synonymous with college Greek Letter Organizations (GLUs—aka Fraternities/Sororities), secret student clubs first prevalent among Ivy League schools and now prevalent at most colleges and universities, including HBCUs. This is a popular image regardless if it is a fair portrayal or not. Membership in these student clubs help establish important connections and contacts that go beyond serving as a source of support and cohesion while attending college. They provide an important link in the Ivy League legacy heritage among generations of families affiliated with their alma mater and are a valuable source of contributions to alum funding drives.

College life, especially for the traditional student attending right out of high school, is also the prime dating scene for these young adults including Dartmouth. Prior to the 1970s, when it was a male-only school, Dartmouth students sought appropriate female companionship from nearby female colleges that also served the privileged elite such as Colby-Sawyer College in New London, New Hampshire. Dartmouth College felt the pressure of social change during the 1970s finally going co-ed in 1972. This change was inevitable as male-only campuses across the nation, including military schools with long traditions, succumbed to public pressure and court orders. Colby-Sawyer College held out longer, only admitting male students in 1989. The co-ed integration movement proved to be a good thing giving that currently colleges and universities generally have a higher female-to-male attendance, including graduate programs. On the other hand, the co-ed mix, especially among youth under age 25, lends itself to highly sexually charged situations that can result in unwanted sexual advances, including rape—a phenomenon common to this age and gender mix regardless if in academia, the military, or similar closed environments. As mentioned in the section of the duty to warn and report, reporting laws relevant to sexual abuse are now compulsory in both state and federal jurisdictions.

The more serious issue is faculty abuse of dependent students, a situation that violates the ethical responsibility of those who violate this trust. Most college students fall within the legally defined status of "adult" and therefore are assumed to hold ultimate responsibility for their behaviors, including consensual sexual activities, even when these behaviors may involve faculty members. Nonetheless, colleges and universities generally frown upon student/faculty intimacy since this behavior tends to erode the social distance and status differential deemed necessary and conducive to a good learning environment. This is especially the case within popular programs with high esteemed faculty whose mentoring is considered a valuable resource for enhancing one's academic and professional career. It is under these circumstances where role expectations are most demanding with greatest emphasis placed on the faculty to maintain the expected professional decorum.

The Dartmouth College sexual harassment suit filed by female graduate students against psychology professors in the Department of Psychological and Brain Sciences (PBS) reflects a problem that seems endemic throughout academia. Not only does it expose the arrogance of entitlement by faculty, including those held in high status by both their academic discipline and the academic institution that benefits from their productivity. The *New Hampshire Union Leader,* the State's largest newspaper, categorized the incident in the Department of PBS as a "21st Century Animal House" drawing reference to the 1978 movie:

> over more than a decade, students filed multiple complains with Dartmouth College administrators alleging sexual harassment and assault by three professors, but nothing was ever done, according to a class action lawsuit filed Thursday in federal court by current and former students.
>
> The seven women each tell a similar story: Three distinguished professors in the Department of Psychological and Brain Sciences—Todd Heatherton, William Kelley and Paul Whalen—were subjecting graduate students to a gauntlet of sexual harassment that included groping, sexting, alcohol-fueled hot tub parties and even rape.
>
> ... Even after several of the women met as a group with Director of Graduate Studies, Thalia Wheatley and Department Chairman Dave Bucci in April 2017 to complain about harassment, administrators did not immediately suspend the men and encouraged the women to continue working with them, according to the lawsuit.
>
> ... The school waited until July 28, 2017, to place Heatherton, Kelley, and Whalen on administrative leave. During that time, Kelley allegedly raped one of the plaintiffs after plying her with alcohol.
>
> After a lengthy internal investigation—which the lawsuit describes as designed to shield the school—Dartmouth allowed Kelley and Whalen to resign and Heatherton to retire.[40]

Dartmouth College reluctantly revoked the offending psychologist's tenure and banned them from campus while strongly denying any administrative failures—a common reframe from organizations attempting to maintain their image and prestige. Any affront to the institution's image could impact grant monies, student enrollment, and even alum gifting. A common practice is to attempt to buy off those making the complaint, or to demonize them, if this option does not work. Another option is to quietly encourage the problem faculty of administrators to pursue employment elsewhere with the promise of a "strong letter of recommendation." This latter process contributes to the "circulation of the elite"—including problem members of the club hence merely transferring these behaviors to another similar venue.[41]

It was a courageous act for these women to file a class-action suit against Dartmouth College given the severe backlash associated with similar attacks on high-powered institutions and individuals. The class-action suit was not for their personal benefit and enrichment. Quite the contrary, it was for all the women subjected to the sexual harassment and demeaning behaviors by powerful faculty who felt immune to any repercussions due to their esteemed academic record of publications, grants, and discipline accolades, let alone their academic pedigree which included top schools in the United States of Canada. The women accusers could have easily avoided the media circus and enjoyed much more profitable outcomes if they agreed to a quiet settlement. But they chose instead to expose this entrenched and protected deviance. Another challenge facing the accusers was the potential loss of their professional career let alone the implied slanderous image that they somehow enticed or provoked their mentors into sexual encounters to advance their own careers (blaming the victim syndrome).

The class-action suit was reduced to 14 million dollars and approved by U.S. District Court Chief Judge Landya McCafferty in January 2020:

> "A class action would achieve an efficient resolution of the class claims, avoiding unnecessary and duplicative litigation for all parties and the judicial system," McCafferty wrote.
>
> The case centers around four claims: Dartmouth violated Title IX by creating a hostile education environment in the Department of Psychological and Brain Sciences; by engaging in gender discrimination; by breaching fiduciary duty; and by being negligent in retention and supervision.
>
> The plaintiffs—current and former students in PBS—alleged in their suit first filed in November 2018 that Dartmouth knew and allowed three tenured professors in the department, Todd Heatherton, William Kelley and Paul Whalen, to create and normalize a sexualized culture, which included a range of behaviors from comments about female students' appearance to sexual assault.
>
> ... Most class members will receive a base payment of $1,000 and be eligible for a supplemental payment based on the effect of the professors' misconduct on their lives.
>
> ... The class, which the parties estimate includes 90 people, is proposed to consist of current and former women graduate students at Dartmouth who were advisees or assistants of one of the three professors between April 1, 2012, and August 31, 2017, and those who co-authored papers with the professors during that time period.[42]

The schizophrenic-like response by the Dartmouth administration is reflected in the seemingly contravening statements directed to the women plaintiffs thanking them for coming forward "to shine a light on the unacceptable environment created by three former faculty members," on the one hand, while lauding the PBS Department Chair, David Bucci, who paid the ultimate price for his department's misadventures via suicide on October 15, 2019. Cited 31 times in the lawsuit for his lack of action and actual harassment of the plaintiffs and continued strong support of this peer and colleagues—Heatherton, Kelley, and Whalen. It is most likely that the sentiments directed toward Dr. Bucci, "the entire Dartmouth community mourns the tragic loss of a remarkable colleague, scholar, teacher, and mentor" holds far more weight than the cleverly coined Campus Culture and Climate Initiative that emerged as a response to the institutionalized sexual harassment situation.[43]

SPS' "Senior Salute"

Another academic sex abuse situation was playing out some 50 miles south of Dartmouth College at SPS—the prestigious Ivy League feeder prep school. Interestingly, both the Dartmouth College plaintiffs and the SPS plaintiff, Chessy Prout, were represented by the same law firm—Sanford Heisler Sharp, LLP. This case had criminal overtones given that the students at SPS range from 14 to 18 with any sexual activity, consensual or otherwise, falls within what is known as "statutory rape" especially if one of the actors is below the age of consent which was 16 in New Hampshire at the time of Owen Labrie's arrest. This case predated that of the Dartmouth College graduate students when it first aired in 2015 headlining that a highly honors senior (6th Form) student, Owen Labrie, enticed a freshman co-ed, Chessy Prout (who rejected the rape-shield protection against naming victim), into a sexual encounter as part of his rite-de-passage from SPS to his entry into Harvard. This rite-de-passage was part of the male elite subculture and, as such, was intended specifically for his male peer audience. Labrie was subsequently convicted on three counts of statutory rape and one count of endangering the welfare of a child, misdemeanors under New Hampshire statutes, and one felony count of using a computer in the commission of his Senior Salute ritual by using a computer to lure a minor for a sexual encounter. Given a relatively light sentence of a year in jail, not prison, and five years' probation, it was the added stigma of having to register as a sex offender that led to the high-profile appeals process that eventually ended in 2020 when all appeals were exhausted.

Again it was the cover-up attempts by an entrenched administration and high-powered elite that led to a more pervasive problem at SPS—that of decades of sex abuse of students by faculty and staff. The aftermath of the unwanted publicity, an embarrassment, to both SPS and the state led to an informal consent decree in lieu of criminal adjudication. Here, the New Hampshire Attorney General (AG) agreed to allow SPS to hire an outside overseer to monitor sexual misconduct at the school. Jeffrey Maher, trained in both criminal justice (MSU/Fitchburg State University) and the law (Massachusetts School of Law), was not of the privileged class (one of the "good ole boys") and therefore had a rocky tenure at SPS. The *Concord Monitor* describes this unique special arrangement between SPS and New Hampshire AG:

> Mather was chosen as the overseer for St. Paul's School at the end of 2018, following a 14-months-long criminal investigation into the school's handling of reported sexual assaults. Rather than pursue charges of child endangerment, a misdemeanor-level offense, the school and state prosecutors reached an agreement that was meant to "facilitate the protection of children at St. Paul's School, and to ensure a system of accountability, oversight, transparency, and training at the school," according to the Attorney General's Office.
>
> Under the agreement, the school agreed to take on Mather for up to five years as an independent compliance overseer who would facilitate student safety, transparency and training at St. Paul's School and make bi-annual reports to the Attorney General.[44]

According to Mather, he received little support from SPS administration. Instead, he felt harassed being forced to filter his reporting through SPS' attorneys and staff. He resigned in October 2020 leading the introduction of the Rape, Abuse & Incest National Network (RAINN) in order for SPS to meet the AG's independent reviewer criterion in order to continue to avoid criminal litigation by the state.

The notoriety of the Labrie case led to the emergence of old cases, some going back six decades with over 60 victims involving 20 named faculty and staff to date. Chessy Prout, with Jenn Abelson of the *Boston Globe*, published a book about her experience—*I Have a Right To: A High School Survivor's Story of Sexual Assault, Justice, and Hope.*[45] Alexander Prout, Chessy's father, addressed the SPS issue in a "My Turn" column for the *Concord Monitor*:

> For more than 150 years, St. Paul's School has enjoyed all the resources New Hampshire has to offer without paying a cent in taxes. Quite the opposite, New Hampshire has given the school, which boasts of an endowment of over $600 million, interest-free loans for the construction of first-class buildings and facilities.

> … Despite those facts, the wealthy and powerful who run this institution have resisted every attempt by New Hampshire officials to ensure that their private, non-profit school protect the children who live and learn on its campus.
>
> St. Paul's believes it is above the law. And for most of its history, the school has escaped legal accountability. With little to no oversight, the school failed to protect its students from sexual assault and harassment and permitted the widespread use of drugs and alcohol by the children of America's elite.
>
> The school's cover-up culture led directly to the rape of my daughter, Chessy Prout, as a part of a tradition of ritualized statutory rape called the senior salute … The school's open contempt for New Hampshire's chief law enforcement officer is not shocking. It views itself as above the law, and it views you and your leaders as rubes. St. Paul School's leaders have bet that Attorney General Gordon MacDonald will do nothing but acquiesce to its demands and, based on his statements following Mr. Maher's resignation, they may be right.[46]

Chessy's assessment differs markedly from that provided by SPS' own account of a pristine, sheltered, and closeted environment. And while this may be the case for many students at SPS, it was not spared the human intrigue inherent within similar institutional settings. Indeed, prestigious academic institutions like SPS may, indeed, be more tolerant of these misdeeds. While more sterile portrayals are presented parroting the official line, best information can be obtained from interviews with the rank-and-file staff who witness these incidents first hand.[47]

The Enshrinement of the Privilege Elite Class via Academic Discourse

America's power elite, and the social structure supporting this system, has been a subject of sociological and social psychological interest since early in the last century up to the present producing such notables as Howard Becker, Emile Durkheim, Michel Foucault, Erich Fromm, Ervin Goffman, Seymore Lipset, Karl Mannheim, Robert K. Merton, C. Wright Mills, Talcott Parsons, W.I. Thomas, and Max Weber, to mention a few. Shamus Rahman Khan cited these scholars (except Fromm and Parsons) in his 2011 book, *Privilege: the Making of an adolescent elite at St. Paul's School*, in an effort to present this work as a scientific ethnomethodological contribution to the discipline of cultural sociology. Khan's book portends to offer a more intimate insight into the everyday life at SPS, going beyond the works of Heckscher in his *A Brief History of St. Paul's School*—an SPS alum like Khan.[48]

Khan's work attempts to depict the socialization/acculturalization process provided by prestigious preparatory schools in reinforcing the youth's, mainly male, privilege status through ritual and customs and how to present and preserve this persona in their adult life. He draws mainly on his own experience as a minority (non-White) student from a privileged wealthy South Asian family background and how SPS teaches people like him to assimilate smoothly into the America predominantly White privileged class. Khan explains the prep school socialization of elitism as follows:

> Through repetition these students gain experience and produce an embodiment of privilege that is not "work" but instead appears a naturalized, innately easy quality. This naturalized privilege … obscures the ways in which privilege is a product of an advantaged social position (attending a $40,000-a-year high school, for one). This aids in both preventing others from displaying the marks of the elite, insofar as the ease is quite difficult to produce, while suggesting that those who are not marked by privilege simply "don't have what it takes."

> We can extend these insights to think about relations among the elite. Being an elite in not a mere possession or something "within" an actor (skills, talents, and human capital); it is an embodied performative act enabled by both possessions and the inscriptions that accompany experiences within elite institutions (schools, clubs, families, networks, etc.).[49]

Khan's book on Privilege is based on his own SPS experience as a student in the 1990s and later as a teacher (Master) teaching while conducting his "participant observation" for his Ph.D. dissertation at the University of Wisconsin–Madison which he received in 2008. Generally speaking, participant observational studies involve someone outside the cultural or subcultural milieu being documented. Reflecting on one's own experience post facto falls more within the realm of literature than social sciences mainly because it is difficult, if not impossible, to divorce one's own emotional involvement from the other subjects under investigation. A classic cultural sociology study is John Dollard's study of the mechanisms of the racial relations in the Jim Crow South prior to World War II.[50] Other notable studies involve youth or motorcycle gangs or bias in law enforcement.

Khan's own elitist background most likely obviated any truly objective insights into gender issues at SPS, despite his attempts at explaining the differential gender socialization process:

> To put it simply, girls have to work harder than boys. Study after study has concluded that girls across the nation have better grades than boys and perform better in college; in no small part this is because they are working harder. But elite colleges are gendered institutions that strive for an equal male-female ration, even though the girls are stronger candidates. Girls at St. Paul's must work harder than boys to find a space within the "girl's pool" of college applicants. Having to work harder makes it harder for girls to display the requisite St. Paul's ease.[51]

Khan's depiction of female students deliberately enticing their male counterparts, including faculty, at SPS is yet another reflection of his own inherent gender bias; one that adheres to the age-old adage of "blaming the victims" aka "they were using their sexuality to provoke us:"

> But the main complaint over seated meals comes from the faculty. The complaint is that girls wear far too little clothing to the meals. Just before I arrived at St. Paul's, the administration changed the rules for girl's dress: they are now required to cover their shoulders, resulting in what was called the "no bare shoulder rule," but many are uncomfortable saying anything to girls about their physical appearance … Senior girls are eighteen years old, and there are several male faculty members who are barely out of college. Girls will often test this tension and push the line of appropriateness … By making faculty uncomfortable, by making the faculty aware that they were (almost) women with bodies like other women in their lives—that they were not children but adults—and by making the faculty aware that we were not infallible, and that at least some of us had inappropriate urges, desires, and thoughts, the girls were able to use their sexuality to subvert authority at the were school.[52]

Khan's dissertation, and subsequent award-winning book, *Privilege* (2011 C. Wright Mills Book Award), failed to disclose the decades of sexual and drug abuse at SPS, events that were made media headlines four years following his book award propelling him to prestigious positions at Columbia University (chair of the Department of Sociology; executive committee, the Institute for Women, Gender, and Sexuality) and his current (2021) transfer to Princeton University. Indeed, Khan downplayed any misbehavior at SPS attributing any such behaviors as falling within the normal pattern of other high school students with no mention of any faculty indiscretions. This sentiment is displayed in footnote 13 to chapter 4 on "Gender and Performance of Privilege":

> Readers may wonder how common homosexuality is at the school, or perhaps how common sex, drinking, or drugs are. Contrary to the image portrayed of elite kids, drug-fueled orgies and wild parties are rare. They never happen on campus—where the risk of getting caught and punished is high. And upon surveying the students about their health, the school essentially found that its students were like other high school student. They were a little more stressed out, which is not surprising. But their rates of sexual activity, of first sexual contact, and of drinking and drugs were the same as those of students across the nation. Students usually leave campus to break the rules. If they do so on campus and are caught, colleges may find out about their transgression, and this could hurt their chances of being accepted. If they do so at home or in a hotel room, colleges are typically never the wiser.[53]

Notes

1 See Durkheim, E. 1949. *The Division of Labor in Society* (Simpson, G., trans.). Glencoe, IL: The Free Press; 1951, *Suicide.* (Spaulding, J.A., & Simpson, G., trans.). Glencoe, IL: The Free Press.

2 *Jane Roe et al. v. Henry Wade, District Attorney of Dallas County (Texas).* 410 U.S. 113; 93 S.Ct. 705; 35 L.Ed. 2d 147; 1973 U.S. LEXIS 159.

3 See French, L.A. 1977. Elitism: Perpetuation Through Incarceration (Cpt. 7), in *Blacks and Criminal Justice* (Owens, C.E., & Bell, J., eds.). Lexington, MA: Lexington Books, pp. 53–66; *Furman v. Georgia,* 408 U.S. 238, 345, 1972; French, L.A. 1978. Incarcerated Black Female: The Case of Social Double Jeopardy. *Journal of Black Studies,* Vol. 8 (3), March, pp. 321–335.

4 See *Education Project in Criminal Justice, Graduate School of Criminal Justice, State University of New York at Albany:* Law Enforcement Assistance Administration (LEAA) (77CD-99-0004; September 1, 1977) & L.A. French, 2018. *The History of Policing America: From Militias and Military to the Law Enforcement of Today.* Latham, MD: Rowman & Littlefield, pp. 164–165.

5 See *Title IX—Safety for Indian Women,* House Resolution 3402, 2013; French, L.A. 2019. Indian Justice in the 21st Century (Cpt. 8), *Routledge Handbook on Native American Justice Issues* (French, L.A., ed.). New York, NY: Routledge/Taylor & Francis, pp. 110–125.

6 See President Trump's Executive Order #13898 (November 28, 2919, *OperationLadyJustice.usdoj.gov.*

7 See Good, H., & Teller, J., 1967. *A History of American Education.* New York, NY: Macmillan; Cremin, L. 1961. *The Transformation of the School.* New York, NY: Vintage.

8 *Ibid.*

9 See Best, J., & Sidwell, R. 1967. *The American Legacy of Learning.* Philadelphia, PA: Lippincott; Potter, R. 1967. *The Stream of American Education.* New York, NY: American Book Company.

10 See Anderson, J.D. 1988. *The Education of Blacks in the South 1860–1935.* Chapel Hill, NC: University of North Carolina Press; Cremin (op. cit. 7); French, L.A. 2014. *Frog Town: Portrait of a French Canadian Parish in New England,* Lanham, MD: Rowman & Littlefield; Fellman, D. 1969. *The Supreme Court and Education.* New York, NY: Teachers College Press & *Servicemen's Readjustment Act of 1944* (chapter 286, 58 Stat. 284).

11 See Pratt, R. 1964. *Battlefield and Classroom* (Utley, R., ed.). New Haven, CT: Yale University Press; French, L.A. 1994. *Psychocultural Change and the American Indian.* New York, NY: Garland.

12 See French, L.A. 1994. *The Winds of Injustice: American Indians and the U.S. Government.* New York, NY: Garland Publishing, Inc.

13 *Ibid.*

14 Costo, R., & Henry, J. 1970. *Textbooks and the American Indian.* San Francisco, CA: Indian Historian Press, p. 247.

15 See *Report on Indian Education,* Task Force Five: Indian Education. Final Report to the American Indian Policy Review Commission. Washington, DC: U.S. Government Printing Office, 1976; *Indian Education Act.* U.S. Statutes at Large 86: 335, 339–343, June 23, 1972; *Indian Self-Determination and Educational Assistance Act.* U.S. Statutes at Large, 58: 2203–14, January 4, 1975.

16 Khan, S.R. 2011. *Privilege: The Making of an Adolescent Elite at St. Paul's School.* Princeton, NJ: Princeton University Press, pp. 32–33.

17 Heckscher, A. 1996. *A Brief History of St. Paul's School, 1856–1996.* Concord, NH: The Board of Trustees of St. Paul's School.

18 *Ibid.*

19 *Ibid.,* pp. 138–139.

20 *Ibid.,* p. 166.

21 See Mead, G.H. 1934. *Mind, Self, and Society.* Chicago, IL: University of Chicago Press.

22 See Kohler, W. 1929. *Gestalt Psychology.* New York, NY: Horace Liveright.

23 See Linton, R. 1936. *The Study of Man.* New York, NY: Appleton-Century Company; Hyman, H., & Singer, E. (eds.). 1968. *Readings in Reference Group Theory and Research.* Glencoe, IL: The Free Press; Durkheim, E. 1951. *Suicide.* Glencoe, IL: The Free Press; Merton, R.K. 1938. Social Structure and Anomie. *American Sociological Review,* Vol. 3, pp. 672–682; Stouffer, S., et al. 1949. *Studies in Social Psychology in World War II: The American Soldier.* Princeton, CT: Princeton University Press.

24 See Weber, M. 1947 (Parsons, T., ed.). *The Theory of Social and Economic Organizations.* Glencoe, IL: The Free Press; Duran, E., & Duran, B. 1995. *Native American Postcolonial Psychology.* Albany, NY: The State University of New York.

25 See Simmel, G. 1955. *Conflict.* (Wolf, K.A., trans.). Glencoe, IL: The Free Press; Coser, L. 1955. *The Functions of Social Conflict.* Glencoe, IL: The Free Press.

26 See French, L.A., & Manzanarez, M. 2004. Culture, Social Status and Education (Part IV), *NAFTA & Neocolonialism: Comparative Criminal, Human & Social Justice,* Lanham, MD: University Press of America, pp. 169–193; The Best Lawyers in the Granite State. *New Hampshire Magazine,* Vol. 34 (#11, November 2020), pp. 61–89.

27 See Cosby, W.H., Jr. 1976. *An Integration of the Visual Media via "Fat Albert and the Cosby Kids" into Elementary School Curriculum as a Teaching Aid and Vehicle to Achieve Increased Learning* (Doctoral Dissertation). Amherst, MA: University of Massachusetts.

28 Leo, J. 1998. Dumbing Down Teachers. *U.S. News & World Report* (August 3), p. 15.

29 See Bear, J., & Bear, M. 2000. *College Degrees by Mail & Internet.* Berkeley, CA: Ten Speed Press; Goldman, C.A., & Massy, W.F. 2001. *The Ph.D. Factory.* Bolton, MA: Anker Publishing Company; *The Bologna Accord: A European Revolution with Global Implications.* www.gmac.com.

30 See APA. 2017. *Ethical Principles of Psychologists and Code of Conduct.* Washington, DC: American Psychological Association; APA 2002. *American Psychologist,* Vol. 57 (12).

31 See Williams, R.B., French, LA., & Ferrell, R. 2006. Observing the Preservation and Decline in Abilities in Dementia. *Psychological Reports,* Vol. 99 (3), pp. 664–670.

32 See French, L.A. 1997. (Book Review). A Criminal Justice Approach. *Criminal Justice Review,* Vol. 22 (1), pp. 95–97.

33 See Bartlett, T. 2019. Florida State University Professor Accused of Fabricating Data—"Cooking the Books." *The Chronicle of Higher Education,* Vol. 66 (4) (September); Walsh, W.B., & Betz, N.E. 1995. *Tests and Assessment.* Englewood Cliffs, NJ: Prentice Hall.

34 See Resendez, A. 2016. Colleras and Epidemics. *The Other Slavery: The Uncovered Story of Indian Enslavement in America.* Boston, MA: Houghton Mifflin Harcourt, pp. 212–217.

35 Tanielian, T., & Jaycox, L.H. (eds.). 2008. *Invisible Wounds of War: Summary and Recommendations for Addressing Psychological and Cognitive Injuries* (Document No. MG-720/1-CCF). Santa Monica, CA: Rand Corporation; French, L.A., & Nikolic-Novakovic, L. 2012. *Was Trauma and Its Aftermath.* Lanham, MD: University Press of America.

36 *Ibid.*

37 Edgerton, J.E., & Campbell, R.J. (eds.). 1994. *American Psychiatry Glossary* (7th ed.). Washington, DC: American Psychiatric Press, Inc., pp. 50, 210.

38 See Coser, L.A. 1977. *Masters of Sociological Thought: Ideas in Historical and Social Context.* New York, NY: Harcourt, Brace and Jovanovich.
39 See Zamudio-Suarez, F. 2018. Former Michigan State President Is Charged With Lying to Police About Larry Nassar. *The Chronicle of Higher Education* (November 20).
40 See Feathers, R. 2018. Former Dartmouth students sue for $70m, Claiming Professors Ran "21st Century Animal House." *New Hampshire Union Leader* (November 15). www.unionleader.com/news/courts/former-dartmouth-students-sue-for-m-claining-professors-ran-st/article; Dandrea A. 2018. Students Accuse Professors of Abuse. *Concord Monitor* (November 16), pp. A1, A6.
41 See Pareto, V. 1935. *The Mind and Society* (Livingston, A., ed.). New York, NY: Harcourt, Brace & Company.
42 See Doyle-Burr, N. 2020. Preliminary Approval on $14M Harassment Settlement. *Concord Monitor* (January 31), p. A4.
43 *Ibid.;* Feather, R., op. cit. 40.
44 See DeWitt, E. 2020. St. Paul's School: RAINN to Review School's Conduct—National Sexual Assault Prevention Group Hired after Compliance Officer Resigned. *Concord, Monitor* (December 23), pp. A1, A2.
45 See Prout, C., & Abelson, J. 2018. *I Have the Right to: A High School's Survivor's Story of Sexual Assault, Justice, and Hope—A Memoir.* New York, NY: Margaret K. McElderry Books/Simon & Schuster.
46 See Prout, A. 2020. St. Paul's School and Accountability. *Concord Monitor* (November 15), p. C2.
47 *Author's disclosure*: Inside knowledge about the functioning of St. Paul's School comes from my, and my wife's, interactions with faculty and staff at SPS starting in 1981. My wife, Nancy, served as office manager for SPS Admissions from 1981 until 1988, and we continued to interact with staff who work there. Knowledge about the student subculture was no secret among staff at SPS—those knew most about the "dirty linen" were those assigned to do the washing.
48 Op. cit. 16, 17.
49 Khan, op. cit. 16, p. 136.
50 See Dollard, J. 1937. *Caste and Class in a Southern Town.* New Haven, CT: Yale University Press.
51 Op. cit. 49, p. 121.
52 *Ibid.,* pp. 122, 123.
53 *Ibid.,* footnote 13 (chapter 4), pp. 218, 219.

8

ETHICS DURING THE TRUMP ERA

Introduction

This chapter will address the ethics relating to three elements of the Trump administration—law and order, border politics, and the COVID response—from the perspective of social justice.

Toward an Understanding of the Mechanism of Social Divisiveness

Lie (a) An assessment of something known or believed by the speaker to be untrue with intent to deceive; (b) an untrue or inaccurate statement that may or may not be believed true by the speaker.[1]

Insurrection An act or instance of revolting against civil authority or an established government.[2]

Clearly, the worldwide coronavirus (COVID-19) will highlight the second decade of the 21st century. Also, the date 01/06/2021 (January 6, 2021) will be remembered as a significant event in the United States, like that of 09/11/2001 (September 11, 2001), in the historical archives of the 21st century. While fresh in our memories at the time of this writing (January 14, 2021—the day following the second impeachment of President Donald J. Trump), historical and political analysis will continue long into the century and beyond. A critical factor here is the pervasive use of lies by a prominent international leader, that of U.S. President, Donald J. Trump (2017–2021), as a propaganda tool and its effect on segments of the population that resulted in marked social divisiveness. The continued use of the "Big Lie" by people in responsible positions draws attention to the ethical responsibilities of people who hold considerable influence over others.

What are the circumstances leading up to an insurrection in an otherwise long-lasting democracy and the role of those in leadership positions? A combined psychological (clinical) and social/cultural assessment is needed in order to better understand the mechanisms of the Trump Era and the political and social divisiveness it created. That said, a demigod can only exploit a social situation that is ripe for social and political confrontation. Racial divisions and the reemergence of radical White supremacy groups festered during the Obama (2009–2017) administration in

DOI: 10.4324/9781003224426-8

reaction by those opposed to having a Black president. Simmering racism had long been evident as a latent functioning of American society, one that waxed and waned from the colonial days, the U.S. Civil War, and circumstances following Reconstruction. Discontent over the Gulf Wars and the pervasive treat of international terrorism ignited by 09/11/01, coupled with the Great Recession, during the George W. Bush (2001–2009) administration provided kinder that was further fueled by the election of America's first Black president—Barak Obama. While the Obama presidency may have set the stage for the insurgence of radical White supremacy and its resulting racism, it was the emergence of Donald J. Trump and his propaganda of mistruths (Big Lie campaign against perceived foes) that led to the attempted insurrection of 01/06/21 as a last ditch effort to overturn the presidential elections and Trump's second impeachment on January 13, 2021.

The psychological factors that help facilitate the era of racism and political divide under the Trump administration include the leader's attributes. Narcissism has long been attributed to Trump's persona. His egotism has classic elements of the *narcissistic personality disorder*:

1. Has a grandiose sense of self-importance (e.g., exaggerates achievements and talents, expects to be recognized as superior without commensurate achievements).
2. Is preoccupied with fantasies of unlimited success, power, brilliance, beauty, or ideal love.
3. Believes that he or she is "special" and unique and can only be understood by, or should associate with, other special or high-status people (or institutions).
4. Requires excessive admiration.
5. Has a sense of entitlement (i.e., unreasonable expectations of especially favorable treatment or automatic compliance with his or her expectations).
6. Is interpersonally exploitative (i.e., takes advantage of others to achieve his or her own ends).
7. Lacks empathy: is unwilling to recognize or identify with the feelings and needs of others.
8. Is often envious of others or believes that others are envious of him or her.
9. Shows arrogant, haughty behaviors or attitudes.[3]

Five of these items determine a diagnosis of the narcissistic personality disorder.

It is not enough for a deluded charismatic individual to hold court within the public arena; he/she needs a susceptible audience in order to acquire an influential power base in order to enact his geopolitical design. Most demigods rely on a hard-core base of cult followers as a sounding board for the more outrageous messages—the Big Lies, told over and over again: "the Media is the Enemy," "opposition political parties and groups are the enemy," "any criticism is a hoax and witch hunt …" The tools for expanding the demigod's influence include social divisions articulated by stereotyping differences like race and ethnicity, gender, nationality, religion, political affiliation, and socioeconomic status. The Big Lie scenario relies on both stereotyping and discrimination with the message constantly repeated, often in simple sound bites ("Make America Great Again," "Lock Her Up," "Stop the Steal") coupled with a constant bombardment dismissive of established entities such as science and news outlets (Fourth Estate) allowing these constantly repeated chants take on a truth ("alternative truths") of their own. Here the attribution bias helps explain the contravening social perceptions emanating from the constant Big Lies told by an influential leader like Presidential Trump.

A compelling question raised by many is how can well-educated individuals be drawn to the Big Lie messages of a demigod—especially those that clearly defy logic? Part of the answer is that our emotional predisposition overrides rationality during times of crisis or normlessness (anomie). During these times, people lose their degree of individuality to a collectivity that provides them with a renewed sense of worth and a defined "out group" as their new enemy. Collective attribution bias helps reinforce the divide between competing groups while providing a rationalization for the respective groups behaviors. Simmel termed this relationship as reciprocal antagonism where each group draws its cohesiveness from the perceived hostilities from the defined, and often, demonized, out-group (e.g., Far Right vs. Far Left political entities). Within this emotionally charged environment, we tend to attribute deliberate hostility to actions of the out-group while justifying similar actions by the in-group. Hence, mass protest by the out-group are labeled "riots" and "mayhem," while similar actions by the in-group are portrayed as the justified action of patriots defending the Constitution.[4] Individuality is often a casualty of mob behavior, especially those incidents ignited by highly charged events, like the killing of unarmed minority members by White law enforcement officers or a charge from a sitting leader that the election was stolen from him. Risky behaviors become contagious during these emotionally charged physical encounters leading to individual behaviors that otherwise would not have occurred.[5]

Ethical Consequences for Pathological Lying

Eric Alterman wrote a book on the history of official deception and its consequences by modern U.S. presidents from Franklin D. Roosevelt to George W. Bush called, *When Presidents Lie.* Published during the George W. Bush administration, an entire new volume could be written solely on the Donald J. Trump administration.[6] Alterman explains the phenomenon of presidential lying as follows:

> In American politics today, the ability to lie convincingly has come to be considered an almost prima facie qualification for holding higher office. Many of the lies that officials tell are obviously harmless. Audiences demand to be flattered and politicians feel compelled to obligate.[7]
>
> In society, as in nature, the failure to appreciate the fact that the behavior of the actors is in part responsible for the environment that will later impinge on them leads observers—and actors as well—to underestimate actors' influence. In terms of the literature of path dependency, we see in a presidential lie the kind of "causal mechanism" that inspires the "inherent logic of events" through which "the impact of decisions (in this case, lies) persists into the present and defines alternatives for the future ... The tendency for leaders to believe their own propaganda over time is one form of what first CIA agents and, later, political sciences have come to call "blowback." One feature of blowback is that its effects are almost always portrayed as unprovoked, often inexplicable actions, when in fact they are typically caused by actions initially taken by the government itself ... But once a president takes it upon himself to lie to the country about important matters, he necessarily creates an independent dynamic that would not otherwise have come about, and we are all the worse for it.[8]

Donald J. Trump's lies went far beyond the harmless platitudes appeasing local audiences. His lies were designed to divide and incite discourse within the American public. According to *The Washington Post*'s "The Fact Checker," the president publically made over 30,000 false or misleading claims starting from his 2016 campaign to his last weeks in office. Incredibly, no one within his party or administration seriously attempted to challenge these mistruths. His perception of "truth" fired up a cross section of Americans who went far beyond White supremacists and other radical racist group—as was evident by his massive rallies including his "call-to-arms" on January 6, 2021, in his last ditch effort to pervert the customary Congressional role of recognizing the already determined Electoral College votes. As the investigation into the planning and execution of this deadly and destructive mob action unfolds, we now see how wide Trump's audience was, including member of Congress, middle-class professional, law enforcement, and current and former members of the military. Included in this mix was a contingency led by U.S. Army Captain Emily Rainey, a "anti-masker" and leader within the Fourth Psychological Operations Group (Army Psychological Warfare) at Fort Bragg in North Carolina. This is interesting given the role previous psychologist played in the Central Intelligence Agency (CIA) torture scandal. Clearly, more needs to be uncovered regarding the planning and intent of the 01/06/2021 to overturn the Biden/Harris election results including alleged plans to arrest and, possibly, execute Vice President Pence and members of Congress. Preliminary evidence, however, was sufficient to warrant an indictment from Congress in the form of an Article of Impeachment.

Article of Impeachment

Articles of Impeachment Against Donald John Trump

{House Resolution 755, One Hundred Sixteenth Congress, First Session}

CONGRESS OF THE UNITED STATES OF AMERICA,
IN THE HOUSE OF REPRESENTATIVES,
December 18, 2019.
RESOLUTION

Resolved, That Donald John Trump, President of the United States, is impeached for high crimes and misdemeanors and that the following articles of impeachment be exhibited to the United States Senate:

Articles of impeachment exhibited by the House of Representatives of the United States of America in the name of itself and of the people of the United States of America, against Donald John Trump, President of the United States of America, in maintenance and support of its impeachment against him for high crimes and misdemeanors.

ARTICLE I: ABUSE OF POWER

The Constitution provides that the House of Representatives "shall have the sole Power of Impeachment" and that the President "shall be removed from Office on Impeachment for, and Conviction of, Treason, Bribery, or other high Crimes and Misdemeanors." In his conduct of the office of President of the United States—and in violation of his constitutional oath faithfully to execute the office of President of the United States and, to the best of his ability, preserve, protect, and defend the Constitution of the United States, and in violation of his constitutional duty to take care that the laws be faithfully executed—Donald J. Trump has abused the powers of the Presidency, in that:

Using the powers of his high office, President Trump solicited the interference of a foreign government, Ukraine, in the 2020 United States Presidential election. He did so through a scheme or course of conduct that included soliciting the Government of Ukraine to publicly announce investigations that would benefit his reelection, harm the election prospects of a political opponent, and influence the 2020 United States Presidential election to his advantage. President Trump also sought to pressure the Government of Ukraine to take these steps by conditioning official United States Government acts of significant value to Ukraine on its public announcement of the investigations. President Trump engaged in this scheme or course of conduct for corrupt purposes in pursuit of personal political benefit. In so doing, President Trump used the powers of the Presidency in a manner that compromised the national security of the United States and undermined the integrity of the United States democratic process. He thus ignored and injured the interests of the Nation.

President Trump engaged in this scheme or course of conduct through the following means:

(1) President Trump—acting both directly and through his agents within and outside the United States Government—corruptly solicited the Government of Ukraine to publicly announce investigations into—
    (A) a political opponent, former Vice President Joseph R. Biden, Jr.; and
    (B) a discredited theory promoted by Russia alleging that Ukraine—rather than Russia—interfered in the 2016 United States Presidential election.
(2) With the same corrupt motives, President Trump—acting both directly and through his agents within and outside the United States Government—conditioned two official acts on the public announcements that he had requested—
    (A) the release of $391 million of United States taxpayer funds that Congress had appropriated on a bipartisan basis for the purpose of providing vital military and security assistance to Ukraine to oppose Russian aggression and which President Trump had ordered suspended; and
    (B) a head of state meeting at the White House, which the President of Ukraine sought to demonstrate continued United States support for the Government of Ukraine in the face of Russian aggression.
(3) Faced with the public revelation of his actions, President Trump ultimately released the military and security assistance to the Government of Ukraine, but has persisted in openly and corruptly urging and soliciting Ukraine to undertake investigations for his personal political benefit. These actions were consistent with President Trump's previous invitations of foreign interference in United States elections.

In all of this, President Trump abused the powers of the Presidency by ignoring and injuring national security and other vital national interests to obtain an improper personal political benefit. He has also betrayed the Nation by abusing his high office to enlist a foreign power in corrupting democratic elections.

Wherefore President Trump, by such conduct, has demonstrated that he will remain a threat to national security and the Constitution if allowed to remain in office, and has acted in a manner grossly incompatible with self-governance and the rule of law. President Trump thus warrants impeachment and trial, removal from office, and disqualification to hold and enjoy any office of honor, trust, or profit under the United States.

ARTICLE II: OBSTRUCTION OF CONGRESS

The Constitution provides that the House of Representatives "shall have the sole Power of Impeachment" and that the President "shall be removed from Office on Impeachment for, and Conviction of, Treason, Bribery, or other high Crimes and Misdemeanors." In his conduct of the office of President of the United States—and in violation of his constitutional oath faithfully to execute the office of President of the United States and, to the best of his ability, preserve, protect, and defend the Constitution of the United States, and in violation of his constitutional duty to take care that the laws be faithfully executed—Donald J. Trump has directed the unprecedented, categorical, and indiscriminate defiance of subpoenas issued by the House of Representatives pursuant to its "sole Power of Impeachment." President Trump has abused the powers of the Presidency in a manner offensive to, and subversive of, the Constitution, in that:

The House of Representatives has engaged in an impeachment inquiry focused on President Trump's corrupt solicitation of the Government of Ukraine to interfere in the 2020 United States Presidential election. As part of this impeachment inquiry, the Committees undertaking the investigation served subpoenas seeking documents and testimony deemed vital to the inquiry from various Executive Branch agencies and offices, and current and former officials.

In response, without lawful cause or excuse, President Trump directed Executive Branch agencies, offices, and officials not to comply with those subpoenas. President Trump thus interposed the powers of the Presidency against the lawful subpoenas of the House of Representatives, and assumed to himself functions and judgments necessary to the exercise of the "sole Power of Impeachment" vested by the Constitution in the House of Representatives.

President Trump abused the powers of his high office through the following means:

(1) Directing the White House to defy a lawful subpoena by withholding the production of documents sought therein by the Committees.
(2) Directing other Executive Branch agencies and offices to defy lawful subpoenas and withhold the production of documents and records from the Committees—in response to which the Department of State,
Office of Management and Budget, Department of Energy, and Department of Defense refused to produce a single document or record.
(3) Directing current and former Executive Branch officials not to cooperate with the Committees—in response to which nine Administration officials defied subpoenas for testimony, namely John Michael "Mick" Mulvaney, Robert B. Blair, John A. Eisenberg, Michael Ellis, Preston Wells Griffith, Russell T. Vought, Michael Duffey, Brian McCormack, and T. Ulrich Brechbuhl.

These actions were consistent with President Trump's previous efforts to undermine United States Government investigations into foreign interference in United States elections.

Through these actions, President Trump sought to arrogate to himself the right to determine the propriety, scope, and nature of an impeachment inquiry into his own conduct, as well as the unilateral prerogative to deny any and all information to the House of Representatives in the exercise of its "sole Power of Impeachment." In the history of the Republic, no President has ever ordered the complete defiance of an impeachment inquiry or sought to obstruct and impede so comprehensively the ability of the House of Representatives to investigate "high Crimes and Misdemeanors." This abuse of office served to cover up the President's own repeated misconduct and to seize and control the power of impeachment—and thus to nullify a vital constitutional safeguard vested solely in the House of Representatives.

In all of this, President Trump has acted in a manner contrary to his trust as President and subversive of constitutional government, to the great prejudice of the cause of law and justice, and to the manifest injury of the people of the United States.

Wherefore, President Trump, by such conduct, has demonstrated that he will remain a threat to the Constitution if allowed to remain in office, and has acted in a manner grossly incompatible with self-governance and the rule of law. President Trump thus warrants impeachment and trial, removal from office, and disqualification to hold and enjoy any office of honor, trust, or profit under the United States.

Speaker of the House of Representatives[9]

Law and Order Under the Trump Administration

Interpretation and implementation of the "Bill of Rights" since the U.S. Congress ratified the first ten Amendments of the U.S. Constitution on December 15, 1791, have varied greatly in America, often reflecting the biases attributed to both politics and public sentiments. History has taught us that judicial interpretations of these rights have favored Whites over the concerns of non-Whites enhancing an environment of White privilege and supremacy. "Constitutional Rights" for non-Whites and females have found formidable roadblocks over the years despite Constitutional, legislative, and judicial interpretations favoring change.

Clearly, the American Constitution, lauded worldwide as the ideal template for democracy, was intended for a select group of White aristocrats. This was the intended audience mentioned in the Preamble:

> We the People of the United States, in order to form a more perfect union, establish justice, insure domestic tranquility, provide for the common defense, promote the general welfare, and secure the blessings of liberty to ourselves and our posterity.[10]

Unfortunately, these principles are still not universally accepted 230 years later. Subtle discrimination has festered since December 1791 relevant to the First, Second, Fourth, Fifth, and Eighth Amendments. Over the years, there have numerous challenges to the interpretation of the First Amendment regarding religion, free speech, the right to assemble, and the press, while Second Amendment Rights to "bear arms" is a more recent controversy given the proliferation of military-style assault rifles and large capacity magazines, let alone silencers and automatic fire conversion devices, among civilians and law enforcement. The Fourth Amendment protection against search and seizure has long been viewed as blatantly racist with minority people more likely to be discriminated against including non-warrant traffic stops (crime of driving while Black, Hispanic, American Indian, Asian), and no-knock, nighttime special weapons and tactics (SWAT) assaults. The Fifth Amendment goes beyond the right to self-incrimination; it also addresses the practice of "law enforcement larceny" whereby property is seized merely on the suspicion of a crime with this "property" going to law enforcement agencies, often with little or no oversight. The internment of suspected terrorist since 09/11/01 without arraignment or adequate defense or other judicial relief is yet another recent questionable Fifth Amendment abuse. People of color, and the poor, are also likely victims of excessive bail and fines and, most importantly, cruel and unusual punishment, conditions prohibited by the Eighth Amendment.[11]

Less subtle discrimination involves the 13th, 14th, 15th, 19th, and 24th Amendments.[12] In 1865, the 13th Amendment was supposed to outlaw slavery and involuntary servitude but added the provision that allowed for the creation of the "Black Codes" and "Pig Laws" the extra-legal foundations of the Jim Crow era including the establishment of the chain gang and long prison sentences for Blacks and other non-Whites in America. Andres Resendez called this *The Other Slavery*:

> In 1865–1866 southern states enacted the infamous Black Codes aimed at restricting the freedom of former slaves. Adopting tried-and-true tactics such as vagrancy laws, convict

> leasing, and debts, White southerners sought to nullify the provisions of the Thirteenth Amendment. The Mississippi legislature was the first to introduce these measures, which were quickly copied, sometimes word for word, in South Carolina, Georgia, Florida, Alabama, Louisiana, and Texas. Mississippi's Vagrant Act of 1865, for instance, required that "all free negroes and mulattoes over the age of eighteen carry written proof of employment." Without such a document, a free Black would be immediately deemed a vagrant and hired out to any White man willing to pay the $50 fine incurred by a convicted vagrant.[13]

Resendez noted that *The Other Slavery*, in violation of the 13th Amendment, had a long history of abuse among other non-Whites including Chinese coolies, Mexican peons, and American Indians with the latter continuing well until the 20th century in places like New Mexico.[14]

Voting rights, due process, and the protection of life, liberty, and property guaranteed by the 14th Amendment are still met with political obstruction notably in the South where State's like Texas allocates a single voting station per county regardless of population density. And, although specifically excluded in the original Amendment, American Indians still face numerous de facto barriers to the civil rights afforded other Americans. The 15th Amendment addressing Black suffrage was evident during the 2020 presidential election when Donald J. Trump attempted to subvert and negate the Black vote in a number of states he won previously in the 2016 election. Even the 19th Amendment, the long fought right for women to vote, had a racist element when Jim Crow laws excluded Blacks, Hispanics, and other minorities of color. A seldom mentioned Civil Rights Amendment was the 24th that outlawed the notorious Southern Black Law of instituting poll taxes as a device to keep Blacks and other minorities from voting. This issue was revisited during the 2020 presidential elections with certain states culling their voting rolls in such a fashion that they excluded mostly impoverished minority communities.[15]

Two players, in addition to President Donald J. Trump, played significant roles in the administration's efforts to return Jim Crow elements into modern American society—Jeff Sessions and Stephen Miller. Jeff Sessions epitomized the neo-Southern conservative being named after Confederate leaders, Jefferson Davis, president of the Confederate States of America, and P.G.T. Beauregard, a leading Confederate Civil War general. His military orientation was via the Boy Scouts of America where he obtained Eagle Scout status. Jeff Sessions, U.S. Senator from Alabama, was confirmed as President Trump's Attorney General (AG) on February 8, 2017, ostensibly rewarding him for his early support and endorsement of Trump's candidacy as well as for his "law and order" stance. One of his first actions to demand the resignation of the pool of U.S. Attorneys appointed by the former Obama administration. This action, in itself, is not controversial and is common practice when a different political party enters the White House. Sessions' more deliberate efforts toward reversing any civil rights progress enacted during the previous administration continued unabated until his forced resignation on November 7, 2018, even under the months of diminished support from President Trump following his decision to recuse himself from the Russian election interference probe into the 2016 presidential elections, a month after taking over the AG's office—an action that clearly infuriated the president.

Some of sessions' first actions were the dismantling of the National Commission on Forensic Science ending Department of Justice (DOJ) review of closed cases, a critical tool in attempts to reverse prejudicial sentencing practices of the past. Along similar lines, Sessions rescinded many guidance documents designed to monitor de facto discrimination within the judiciary relevant to excessive fees and bail for poor and minority defendants and providing accommodations for the developmentally disabled, among other guidance documents. Similarly, the AG dismantled the numerous "consent decrees" and DOJ investigations of police brutality and excessive force, especially by White police against minority suspects. Sessions went further in his efforts to overturn progressive sentencing disparities based on race and class enacted by the Obama administration by ordering federal prosecutors with the DOJ to seek the maximum criminal penalty for drug cases, essentially reenacting the previous maximum sentences formula stemming back to the Reagan era that led to America's embarrassing mass incarceration debacle. Accordingly, Sessions opposed the Sentencing Reform and Corrections Act and, instead, ordered federal prosecutors to seek the death penalty for major drug dealer, a questionable action given the restrictions for capital punishment outlined in the 1976 U.S. Supreme Court (USSC) on capital cases.[16]

Sessions' replacement, William Barr who previously served in the AG position under George H.W. Bush (1989–1993), continued the conservative agenda he inherited. William Barr had the added advantage of strong support from President Trump. This support stemmed from the fact that the new AG seemingly placed the president's interest over that of the objectivity of the DOJ and its mandate for neutrality, essentially serving as Trump's personal lawyer. Most significantly, Barr acted on Sessions' death penalty initiative. Both Sessions and Barr trace their interest in the federal death sentence to the Reagan administration where George H.W. Bush served as vice president. As early as 1992, AG Barr advocated the death penalty as part of recommendations in order to combat violent crimes arguing that it acts as a deterrent while incapacitating offenders from killing again. Barr also noted that the death sentence serves the important societal goal of "just retribution" reaffirming society's "moral outrage" toward murderers.[17]

Marl Silk, in the Politics and Society News of *America: The Jesuit Review*, noted that: "While President Trump is notorious for advocating the death penalty in certain situations, he did not put capital punishment on his agenda as presidential candidate or president. There's every reason to believe that the agenda was Barr's own."[18] Silk brings up Pope Francis statement that the death penalty is "inadmissible," regardless of the offense hence making Barr a Catholic hypocrite despite his being awarded the "Christifideles Laici" (Christ's Lay Faithful Award) last year following his presentation at the National Catholic Prayer Breakfast. Silk also cites a 1998 article by now-Associate Supreme Court Justice, Amy Coney Barrett, that stated that Catholic judges were obligated by oath and profession to recuse themselves from presiding over death penalty cases, something neither she or some of her colleagues did in the recent USSC decision allowing the continuation of Trump's death sentence spree. These decisions regarding the death penalty also clouds the Catholic Church's strong stance against abortion.[19] Clearly, religion, notably "conservative theology," plays a significant role in these "life-and-death" debates rather it be Sessions Southern Methodist, Barr's Roman Catholicism, or the influence of the Southern Baptists. Collectively, these Christian conservatives contributed to Donald J. Trump's base and continued to do so. This same base has contributed to, and resisted efforts to, confront, institutional/systemic racism in American society. This phenomenon represents the modern continuation of the earlier tenths of eugenics as the foundation of White supremacy—the self-righteous stance of "life at conception" but death for the so-called defectives (people of color, poor, minority ethnics, etc.). This argument is evident in the recent divisions within the Southern Baptist Convention (SBC) and Black member churches where the latter are challenging the continued doctrine of segregation and racism being promoted at SBC seminaries in their efforts to demonize the "Black Lives Matter" movement. The sentiment of many Black pastors was expressed in January 2021 by the Reverend Charles Dates of the Progressive Baptist Church of Chicago: "When did the theological architects of American slavery develop the moral character to tell the church how it should discuss and discern racism."[20]

President Trump did nothing to stop the continuation of Barr's death sentence parade even following his resignation. Indeed, Trump went on to pardon or commute a number of former military (Army) personnel, Border Patrol agents, or Blackwater contractors convicted of murder under federal jurisdictions, including Michael Behenna for killing an unarmed Iraqi man; Clint

Lorance, for ordering the killing of unarmed Afghanistan civilians; Mathew Golsteyn, convicted of killing suspected bomb-maker in Afghanistan; Nicholas Slatten, Paul Slough, Evan Liberty, and Dustin Heard, all convicted for the 2007 massacre of unarmed civilians, including children, in Nisour Square in Baghad; and Border Patrol agents Ignacio Ramos and Jose Compcon for killing suspected drug smugglers in 2009 (their sentences were previously commuted by President George W. Bush). The long-held argument that capital punishment is a deterrent falls short when the most recent data from Center for Disease Control and Prevention (CDC), National Center for Health Statistics records 19,141 homicide in the United States for 2019 (a 5.8 rate among 100,000 population) with 14,414 of these deaths caused by firearms. The question is who is to be selected for execution from this massive cohort?[21]

It is difficult to adequately measure the degree of brutality involved in homicide cases, rather it be a public execution by a policeman's knee on someone's neck or being strangled and then having a live fetus removed, or to sufficiently measure the degree of suffering of the victim's relatives. Impulsive acts of violence do not generally rise to the long-held standard of *mens rea*—or competency and willful intent. Mens rea, inherited from British common laws, has been the dejure standard for felonies in America from colonial times and especially for the death sentence. However, the great divide between "procedural (dejure) justice"—that based on judicial ideals, and "distributive (de facto) justice"—the actual practice of judicial ideals, is most evident in capital punishment cases. Historically, this divide was illustrated by Jim Crow, eugenics-based justice until USSC intervention in the early 1970s. The racial/class disparity was augmented by clinical petitions to the USSC over the next 30 years as more became known about human neurophysiology. A major medical awareness was that individuals, regardless of race/ethnicity or gender, were not fully capable of "rational" actions until maximum skeletal and neurological growth was reached at a minimum age of about 18 for most. This was due to an underdeveloped frontal lobe, the neurological region responsible for "rational thought" has not been fully insulated (myelinated) making the individual prone to impulsive dysregulation. The American Psychological Association (APA) played a significant role in support of milestone clinical cases—the 2002 *Atkins v. Virginia* and 2005 *Roper v. Simmons* USSC cases—among others. The former disallowed the execution of the mentally retarded, a practice extending back to the early 20th-century eugenics movement, while the latter prohibited the death sentence for crimes, including homicide, committed by anyone under age 18. These critical clinical/legal cases are articulated by Associate Supreme Court Justice, Honorable Sonia Sotomayor in her dissent to the USSC's refusal to stop Trump's federal executions.[22]

Justice Sotomayor's Dissent

> TO VACATE STAY [January 15, 2021] JUSTICE SOTOMAYOR, dissenting.
>
> After seventeen years without a single federal execution, the Government has executed twelve people since July. They are Daniel Lee, Wesley Purkey, Dustin Honken, Lezmond Mitchell, Keith Nelson, William LeCroy Jr., Christopher Vialva, Orlando Hall, Brandon Bernard, Alfred Bourgeois, Lisa Montgomery, and, just last night, Corey Johnson. Today, Dustin Higgs will become the thirteenth. To put that in historical context, the Federal Government will have executed more than three times as many people in the last six months than it had in the previous six decades.
>
> This unprecedented rush of federal executions has predictably given rise to many difficult legal disputes. One source of confusion has been the Federal Death Penalty Act (FDPA), which Congress enacted in 1994 to guide the imposition and implementation of federal death sentences. Pub. L. No. 103–322, Tit. VI, §60002(a), 108 Stat. 1959 (codified as amended

at 18 U. S. C. §3591 et seq.). Prior to last July, the Federal Government had executed just three people since the enactment of the FDPA, two in 2001 and one in 2003. Many questions about the FDPA remain unanswered.

Another source of uncertainty has been the Department of Justice's (DOJ) announcement of a new execution protocol (the 2019 Protocol). Whereas the previous protocol prescribed a three-drug cocktail for use in executions, the 2019 Protocol calls for a single drug: pentobarbital. Difficulty in obtaining the required drugs had contributed to the Government's nearly two-decade hiatus in carrying out executions. The Government surely knew the 2019 Protocol would face further litigation.

Against this backdrop of deep legal uncertainty, the DOJ did not tread carefully. Simultaneous with the announcement of the 2019 Protocol, it scheduled five executions; eight would follow in the months to come. This rapid pace required those facing execution to fast-track challenges to their sentences. Rather than permit an orderly resolution of these suits, the Government consistently refused to postpone executions and sought emergency relief to proceed before courts had meaningful opportunities to determine if the executions were legal.

Throughout this expedited spree of executions, this Court has consistently rejected inmates' credible claims for relief. The Court has even intervened to lift stays of execution that lower courts put in place, thereby ensuring those prisoners' challenges would never receive a meaningful airing. The Court made these weighty decisions in response to emergency applications, with little opportunity for proper briefing and consideration, often in just a few short days or even hours. Very few of these decisions offered any public explanation for their rationale.

This is not justice. After waiting almost two decades to resume federal executions, the Government should have proceeded with some measure of restraint to ensure it did so lawfully. When it did not, this Court should have. It has not. Because the Court continues this pattern today, I dissent.

The Government will execute Dustin Higgs tonight. In 2001, the United States District Court for the District of Maryland sentenced Higgs to death for his involvement in the kidnapping and killing of three people. The FDPA requires that a federal death sentence be "implement[ed]" "in the manner prescribed by the law of the State in which the sentence is imposed." 18 U. S. C. §3596(a). If that State does not allow the death penalty, the FDPA directs courts to designate an alternate State that does. Executions were legal in Maryland in 2001, so the District Court's Judgment and Order did not designate an alternate State. See App. to Pet. for Cert. 18a–21a. Maryland has since abolished the death penalty, however, so the Government cannot implement the death sentence in accordance with Maryland law as the FDPA requires.

In August 2020, the Government asked the District Court to amend its Judgment and Order to designate Indiana, where Higgs and all other federal death-row prisoners are imprisoned, as the alternate State. Consistent with its current practice, the Government set an execution date before the District Court could rule. The District Court denied the Government's motion, holding that the court had no authority to modify its original judgment. See 2020 WL 7707165, *4 (D Md., Dec. 29, 2020) ("The Government's initial, extraordinary request that the Court amend its original judgment and sentence is something that the Court plainly cannot do"). The Government appealed to the Court of Appeals for the Fourth Circuit, which scheduled oral argument for January 27, 2021. Unwilling to wait, the Government asks this Court to grant certiorari and summarily reverse the District

Court without normal briefing or argument, and direct the District Court to designate Indiana as the Government requested.

Ordinarily, this Court grants petitions for certiorari before judgment only "upon a showing that the case is of such imperative public importance as to justify deviation from normal appellate practice and to require immediate determination in this Court." This Court's Rule 11. The Government falls far short of meeting this strict standard. Whether district courts can amend final orders and judgments in this situation is an open and novel question on which none of the courts of appeals have spoken. After failing to act since Higgs' sentence was imposed in 2001, the Government gives no compelling reason why it suddenly cannot wait a few weeks while courts give his claim the consideration it deserves. Certainly, there is no "imperative public importance" behind the Government's request. I would deny the Government's petition.

Sadly, it is not surprising that the Court grants this extraordinary request. Over the past six months, this Court has repeatedly sidestepped its usual deliberative processes, often at the Government's request, allowing it to push forward with an unprecedented, breakneck timetable of executions. With due judicial consideration, some of the Government's arguments may have prevailed and some or even many of these executions may have ultimately been allowed to proceed. Others may not have been. Either way, the Court should not have sanctioned these executions without resolving these critical issues. The stakes were simply too high.

Even after thirteen federal executions in six months, basic, recurring questions about the FDPA and the 2019 Protocol remain unanswered. For example, what does it mean to "implement" a federal death sentence "in the manner prescribed by the law of the State"? 18 U. S. C. §3596(a). Answers run the gamut. Some judges believe the FDPA merely requires following the State's "top-line choice Cite as among execution methods such as hanging, electrocution, or lethal injection." In re Fed. Bureau of Prisons' Execution Protocol Cases, 955 F. 3d 106, 113 (CADC 2020) (Execution Protocol Cases I) (Katsas, J., concurring). Others read the FDPA to incorporate nearly all state execution protocols, including those details that precede the execution itself. See Order in In re Fed. Bureau of Prisons' Execution Protocol Cases, No. 20–5361, at 4–5 (CADC, Dec. 10, 2020) (en banc) (per curiam) (Execution Protocol Cases II) (Wilkins, J., dissenting); see also Execution Protocol Cases I, 955 F. 3d, at 149, 151 (Tatel, J., dissenting). This Court has yet to say which interpretation is correct. See Mitchell v. United States, 591 U. S. ___, ___ (2020) respecting denial of application for stay) (slip op., at 2) (calling for the Court to "address this issue in an appropriate case"). Worse, the Court has actively prevented lower courts from providing definitive answers themselves. Just four days ago, the D. C. Circuit granted Lisa Montgomery a stay of her execution so it could decide this issue en banc. See Order in Montgomery v. Rosen, No. 21–5001 (Jan. 11, 2011) (en banc). This Court vacated that stay without explanation. Montgomery was executed hours later.

Another outstanding question concerns the FDPA's provision that "[a] sentence of death shall not be carried out upon a person who is [intellectually disabled]." 18 U. S. C. §3596(c). Alfred Bourgeois and Corey Johnson presented substantial evidence that they were intellectually disabled under modern diagnostic standards. Lower courts, however, held that these inmates were barred from challenging their executions on this ground because they had previously been denied relief under outdated diagnostic standards. See 28 U. S. C. §2255(h). Yet there are compelling reasons to believe that the FDPA directs courts to evaluate intellectual disability based on the standards prevailing at the time of the execution. See Bourgeois

v. Watson, 592 U. S. ___, ___–___ (2020) (SOTOMAYOR, J., dissenting from denial of certiorari and application for stay) (slip op., at 2–4); Order in United States v. Johnson, No. 20–15, pp. 4–5 (CA4, Jan. 14, 2021) (Wynn, J., dissenting from denial of rehearing en banc); Order in United States v. Johnson, No. 20–15, p. 7 (CA4, Jan. 12, 2021) (Motz, J., concurring in part in denial of stay). On that view, prior proceedings relying on obsolete medical standards do not preclude consideration of whether an individual "is" intellectually disabled at the time of his execution. 18 U. S. C. §3596(c). This Court should have answered this consequential question before allowing the Government to execute Bourgeois and Johnson. Their executions may well have been illegal. The Court has also allowed executions to proceed in the face of significant challenges to the 2019 Protocol's method of execution. A federal district court found that Daniel Lee, Wesley Purkey, and Keith Nelson were likely to succeed in showing that the 2019 Protocol violates the Eighth Amendment because pentobarbital causes fluid to rapidly accumulate in the lungs, resulting in "extreme pain, terror and panic." See In re Federal Bureau of Prisons' Execution Protocol Cases, 471 F. Supp. 3d 209, 218–219 (DC 2020). Accordingly, the District Court preliminarily enjoined executions under the 2019 Protocol. Id., at 225. This Court vacated the injunction and allowed the executions to move forward, concluding that the Government's "competing expert testimony" rendered a "last-minute" stay inappropriate. Barr v. Lee, 591 U. S. ___, ___ (2020) (per curiam) (slip Cite as: 592 U. S. ____ (2021) 7 SOTOMAYOR, J., dissenting op., at 3). Lee and Purkey, however, did not file their claims at the last minute. They did so shortly after the DOJ announced the new protocol and scheduled their executions. Nelson raised his claim before his execution was even announced. It was the Government, not the inmates, who charged ahead with conducting executions under the challenged protocol, creating an "artificial claim of urgency to truncate ordinary procedures of judicial review." Id., at ___ (SOTOMAYOR, J., dissenting) (slip op., at 1). The Court condoned the Government's tactics and granted a stay.

This Court repeated this error just this week. On December 16, 2020, both Corey Johnson and Dustin Higgs tested positive for COVID–19. They quickly moved to enjoin their executions, arguing that lung damage caused by the virus substantially increased the likelihood they would suffer torturous effects if executed with pentobarbital. The District Court held an evidentiary proceeding and agreed. In re Federal Bureau of Prisons' Execution Protocol Cases, ___ F. Supp. 3d ___, ___–___, 2021 WL 106576, *5–*9 (DDC, Jan. 12, 2021). This time, the Court of Appeals stayed the injunction, relying on this Court's flawed decision in Lee. Order in Roane v. Rosen, No. 21–5004, p. 4 (CADC, Jan. 13, 2021) (Katsas, J., concurring). This Court left that ruling in place, again allowing these executions to proceed despite the District Court's careful fact-finding and the risk of needless and significant pain.

The issues left unresolved during this saga do not end with the FDPA and 2019 Protocol. Many other challenges deserved this Court's review. None were granted. While I cannot catalogue all these claims here, some particularly troubling ones bear mention. Consider again Corey Johnson. In addition to the claim already discussed, Johnson sought a reduction of his death sentence under the First Step Act of 2018, Pub. L. No. 115–8 UNITED STATES v. HIGGS SOTOMAYOR, J., dissenting 391, 132 Stat. 5194. The District Court denied Johnson's motion, concluding that his death sentence was for a crime that was not a "covered offense." See United States v. Johnson, No. 3:92–cr–68 (ED Va., Nov. 19, 2020). The Fourth Circuit denied a stay pending appeal. See Order in United States v. Johnson, Nos. 20–15, 21–1, 21–2 (Jan. 12, 2021). Judge Motz dissented from the denial of stay based on Johnson's First Step Act claim, explaining that the application of the definition of "covered offense""present[s] difficult and important issues necessitating adequate consideration by this court." Id., at 9.

Judge Motz was right. In fact, the courts of appeals have divided on the proper way to interpret the statute's "covered offense" definition.2 When Johnson sought a stay, this Court had already granted certiorari to resolve a split implicating this question. See Pet. for Cert. in No. 20-5904. Rather than granting Johnson a stay and holding his case for reconsideration in light of this, the Court allowed the Government to execute Johnson without any appellate court ruling on the merits of his claims. Consider next Brandon Bernard. Bernard, who was only eighteen when he committed the crimes for which he was executed, raised credible allegations that the Government secured his death sentence by withholding exculpatory evidence and eliciting knowingly false testimony in violation of Brady v. Maryland, 373 U. S. 83 (1963), and Napue v. Illinois, 360 U. S. 264 (1959). But Bernard never received consideration of those claims on the merits. Instead, the Court of Appeals for the Fifth Circuit held that, even though Bernard could not have known about the suppressed evidence when he filed his first habeas petition those claims were subject to the general bar on second-or successive habeas petitions. United States v. Bernard, 820 Fed. Appx. 309 (2020) (per curiam); see also 28 U. S. C. §2255(h)(1).

As Bernard correctly argued, the Fifth Circuit's ruling cannot be reconciled with this Court's decision in Panetti v. Quarterman, 551 U. S. 930 (2007), which held that the bar on second-or-successive petitions does not apply to claims that were not ripe when an inmate filed his first-in-time petition. Bernard v. United States, 592 U. S. ___, ___ (2020) (SOTOMAYOR, J., dissenting) (slip op., at 4). Indeed, the Fifth Circuit's rule makes no sense, as it "perversely rewards the Government for keeping exculpatory information secret until after an inmate's first habeas petition has been resolved." Id., at ___ (slip op., at 5). Unmoved, this Court denied Bernard's petition for a writ of certiorari and application for a stay, leaving this dangerous precedent in place and, again, condoning the Government's tactics.

Finally, consider Wesley Purkey and Lisa Montgomery, whose executions this Court allowed even though the district courts concluded they were likely to succeed in showing that they had no "'rational understanding' of why the State want[ed] to execute [them]." See Madison v. Alabama, 586 U. S. ___, ___ (2019) (slip op., at 17) (quoting Panetti, 551 U.S., at 958). Wesley Purkey suffered from Alzheimer's disease. Thousands of pages of evidence suggested that he earnestly and steadfastly believed that the Government planned to execute him in retaliation for his "protracted jailhouse lawyering" to expose prison abuses. Electronic Case Filing in No. 1:19–cv–3570 (DDC), Doc. 1-18, p. 12; see also Barr v. Purkey, 591 U. S ___, ___–___ (2020) (SOTOMAYOR, J., dissenting) (slip op., at 4–5). The District Court therefore preliminarily enjoined Purkey's execution. Skipping over the Court of Appeals, the Government sought immediate relief from this Court, which vacated the injunction without comment.

Lisa Montgomery likewise made a "substantial threshold showing" to the District Court that she was incompetent to be executed. See Electronic Case Filing in No. 2:21–cv–20 (SD Ind.), Doc. 17, p. 15. Based on expert evidence that Montgomery was experiencing a dissociative psychotic state, the District Court concluded that her "current mental state is so divorced from reality that she cannot rationally understand the government's rationale for her execution." Id., at 18. These findings with respect to Purkey and Montgomery raised significant questions as to whether their executions comported with the Constitution. We will never have definitive answers to those questions because this Court sanctioned their executions anyway.

There is no matter as "grave as the determination of whether a human life should be taken or spared." Gregg v. Georgia, 428 U. S. 153, 189 (1976) (opinion of Stewart, Powell, and Stevens, JJ.). That decision is not something to be rushed or taken lightly; there can be no "justice on the fly" in matters of life and death. See Nken v. Holder, 556 U. S. 418, 427 (2009). Yet the Court has allowed the United States to execute thirteen people in six months under a statutory scheme and regulatory protocol that have received inadequate scrutiny, without resolving the serious claims the condemned individuals raised. Those whom the Government executed during this endeavor deserved more from this Court. I respectfully dissent.[23]

Border Justice

One of President Trump's rallying cries was constructing a wall along the U.S./Mexico border. Jeff Sessions and his ally, Stephen Miller, played a significant role in stirring up anti-Mexican vitriolic sentiments among Trump's White supporters. One of Sessions' earliest actions as U.S. AG was to single out so-called sanctuary cities—those municipalities that refused to enforce federal laws against "illegal immigrants." On March 27, 2017, the AG attempted to punish these sanctuary cities by withholding funding for federal programs. Letters were sent out in April of that year to nine sanctuary cities giving them a DOJ compliance deadline of June 30. This effort was challenged in the courts and never fully implemented. However, both Sessions and Miller played a significant role in the Trump administration's family separation project. This cruel policy criminalized people seeking asylum in the United States by detaining those who did not run the gauntlet of newly imposed hurdles and restrictions designed to stall and deny entry to those arriving at the U.S./Mexico border. Miller continued to foster the racism philosophy shared with his mentors, Sessions and Steve Bannon, that people of color were biologically inferior and more prone to violence mimicking the rationale of the earlier eugenics movement in the United States that fueled systemic racism and support for the Jim Crow era.[24]

This philosophy behind the "Build the Wall" policy became evident in President Trump's first presidential address to the nation on January 8, 2019.

President Trump's January 2019 "Border Wall" Address to the Nation

THE PRESIDENT: My fellow Americans: Tonight, I am speaking to you because there is a growing humanitarian and security crisis at our southern border.

Every day, Customs and Border Patrol Agents encounter thousands of illegal immigrants trying to enter our country. We are out of space to hold them, and we have no way to promptly return them back home to their country.

America proudly welcomes millions of lawful immigrants who enrich our society and contribute to our nation. But all Americans are hurt by uncontrolled, illegal migration. It strains public resources and drives down jobs and wages. Among those hardest hit are African Americans and Hispanic Americans.

Our southern border is a pipeline for vast quantities of illegal drugs, including meth, heroin, cocaine, and fentanyl. Every week, 300 of our citizens are killed by heroin alone, 90 percent of which floods across our southern border. More Americans will die from drugs this year than were killed in the entire Vietnam War.

In the last two years, ICE officers made 266,000 arrests of aliens with criminal records, including those charged or convicted of 100,000 assaults, 30,000 sex crimes, and 4,000 violent killings. Over the years, thousands of Americans have been brutally killed by those who illegally entered our country, and thousands more lives will be lost if we don't act now.

This is a humanitarian crisis—a crisis of the heart and a crisis of the soul.

Last month, 20,000 migrant children were illegally brought into the United States—a dramatic increase. These children are used as human pawns by vicious coyotes and ruthless gangs. One in three women are sexually assaulted on the dangerous trek up through Mexico. Women and children are the biggest victims, by far, of our broken system.

This is the tragic reality of illegal immigration on our southern border. This is the cycle of human suffering that I am determined to end.

My administration has presented Congress with a detailed proposal to secure the border and stop the criminal gangs, drug smugglers, and human traffickers. It's a tremendous problem. Our proposal was developed by law enforcement professionals and border agents at the Department of Homeland Security. These are the resources they have requested to properly perform their mission and keep America safe. In fact, safer than ever before.

Furthermore, we have asked Congress to close border security loopholes so that illegal immigrant children can be safely and humanely returned home.

Finally, as part of an overall approach to border security, law enforcement professionals have requested $5.7 billion for a physical barrier. At the request of Democrats, it will be a steel barrier rather than a concrete wall. This barrier is absolutely critical to border security. It's also what our professionals at the border want and need. This is just common sense.

The border wall would very quickly pay for itself. The cost of illegal drugs exceeds $500 billion a year—vastly more than the $5.7 billion we have requested from Congress. The wall will also be paid for, indirectly, by the great new trade deal we have made with Mexico.

Senator Chuck Schumer—who you will be hearing from later tonight—has repeatedly supported a physical barrier in the past, along with many other Democrats. They changed their mind only after I was elected President.

Democrats in Congress have refused to acknowledge the crisis. And they have refused to provide our brave border agents with the tools they desperately need to protect our families and our nation.

The federal government remains shut down for one reason and one reason only: because Democrats will not fund border security.

My administration is doing everything in our power to help those impacted by the situation. But the only solution is for Democrats to pass a spending bill that defends our borders and re-opens the government.

This situation could be solved in a 45-minutes meeting. I have invited Congressional leadership to the White House tomorrow to get his done. Hopefully, we can rise above partisan politics in order to support national security.

Some have suggested a barrier is immoral. Then why do wealthy politicians build walls, fences, and gates around their homes? They don't build walls because they hate people on the outside, but because they love the people on the inside. The only thing that is immoral is the politicians to do nothing and continue to allow more innocent people to be so horribly victimized.

America's heart broke the day after Christmas when a young police officer in California was savagely murdered in cold blood by an illegal alien, who just came across the border. The life of an American hero was stolen by someone who no right to be in our country.

Day after day, precious lives are cut short by those who have violated our borders. In California, an Air Force veteran was raped, murdered, and beaten to death with a hammer by an illegal alien with a long criminal history. In Georgia, an illegal alien was recently charged with murder for killing, beheading, and dismembering his neighbor. In Maryland, MS-13 gang members who arrived in the United States as unaccompanied minors were arrested and charged last year after viciously stabbing and beating a 16-year-old girl.

Over the last several years, I've met with dozens of families whose loved ones were stolen by illegal immigration. I've held the hands of the weeping mothers and embraced the grief-stricken fathers. So sad. So terrible. I will never forget the pain in their eyes, the tremble in their voices, and the sadness gripping their souls.

How much more American blood must be shed before Congress does it job?

To those who reuse to compromise in the name of border security, I would ask:

> Imagine if it was your child, your husband, or your wife whose life was so cruelly shattered and totally broken?
>
> To every member of Congress: Pass a bill that ends this crisis.
>
> To every citizen: Call Congress and tell them to finally, after all of these decades, secure our border.

This is a choice between right and wrong, justice and injustice. This is about whether we fulfill our sacred duty to the American citizens we serve.

When I took the Oath of Office, I swore to protect our country. And that is what I will always do, so help me God.

Thank you and goodnight.[25]

French and Manzanarez's assessment of President Trump's address articulates the fallacy of his argument and its race-baiting allure in their 2019 book, *Borders and Immigration*:

> President Trump's prime-time speech to the nation has hallmarks of fear-mongering by misusing data in order to create a sense of security emergency and impending crisis which does not exist while, at the same time, demonizing Hispanics, Indians, and Mestizos seeking asylum in the United States which is a right under international law of which America is a co-signee. The Trump administration has deliberately created a self-fulfilling prophecy by orchestrating the "humanitarian crisis" alluded to in the presidential address. This crisis was created by systematically reducing the number of legitimate points of entry as well as limiting the availability of immigration judges needed to hear asylum appeals. These actions caused most potential applicants to attempt other entry points and, by doing so, labeled these individuals as entering illegally, which the administration has deemed a criminal offense. Furthermore, President Trump fails to recognize the legitimacy of those seeking asylum by his administration's attempts to return these people, including children, "back home." The assumption given in the speech is that most, if not all, of those seeking entry into the United States are not eligible or welcomed.
>
> The President also misrepresents marketplace demands, first by stating that these migrants, if allowed to enter the United States, will put a strain on public resources and drive down jobs and wages, especially for other minorities in America (African Americans and Hispanic Americans). This is a weak argument given America's booming economy and the fact that Mexicans and Central Americans have traditionally taken on jobs that are unpopular among U.S. citizens regardless of race or ethnicity. Another market fallacy is the impression that a secure wall will end America's drug dependency. Even if a barrier was erected along the entire 1,933-mile border, it would not, in itself, adequately address the supply issue, let alone the

> demand for these substances within American society. The greatest fallacy in the president's speech, however, is his attempt to paint the majority of those seeking entry into the United States along the southern border as a dangerous and violent race of people. This is a popular propaganda tacit based on the "confirmation bias"—whereby taking a few unrepresentative examples out of context and attributing these to the entire class of people.[26]

The Southern Poverty Law Center (SPLC) has led the way in exposing the racist trend within the Trump administration noting that the president is responsible for putting the White nationalist agenda into action by surrounding himself with far-right ideologues like Jeff Session and Stephen Miller. In its 2018 "Year-End Report," the SPLC called up President Trump on promoting his "Big Lie" linking Hispanic and Indigenous asylum seekers as "animals" and "criminals."[27] The SPLC notes that President Trump's immigration policy is greatly influenced by false narratives presented by the Center for Immigration Studies (CIS) and other anti-immigration hate groups. Detaining asylum seekers, punishing sanctuary cities, and enlisting local law enforcement agencies in the enforcement of federal immigration roundups are policies that come straight from the CIS playbook. Accordingly, Stephen Miller and the CIS also played a major role in President Trump's Muslim ban.[28]

The APA, in early 2020, called for the halt to the sharing of confidential therapy session, of underage asylum detainees, between the Office of Refugee Resettlement (ORR) and the U.S. Immigration and Customs Enforcement (ICE) as justification for continued detainment and/or subsequent deportment. APA head, Arthur C. Evans, Jr., called the sharing of confidential information gleaned from compulsory therapy sessions as unethical and in violation of prevailing ethical standards regarding client, notably that involving "minors"—a process he termed "weaponizing therapy sessions." Here, confidential therapy notes, taken without the client's knowledge as to their use and without legal representation or adequate translation, provided by ORR are used by ICE before immigration hearings as evidence for not providing asylum and for continued detainment and eventual deportation.[29]

In November 2020, U.S. District Judge Emmet Sullivan issued a preliminary injunction ordering the Trump administration from deporting minors before they could request asylum or other protection under federal law. Norman Merchant noted in this report that the Trump administration had expelled at least 200,000 people since March 2020, including 8,800 unaccompanied children or youth, using the coronavirus as justification for this action. The Judge's action only applies to unaccompanied children and youth. The administration's action was initiated by Vice President Mike Pence when he directed the CDC to use its emergency powers to seal the U.S. borders even though the science did not support his contention posed a viable threat to Border Patrol, ICE, or anyone else whose job it was to accommodate and process those seeking asylum. Olivia Troye, a former top aide to the vice president who resigned over the order, stated that this order was aggressively pushed by Stephen Miller.[30]

The Trump Administration's Family Separation Policy

Perhaps the most heartless of Trump's border policies was the "Family Separation" program devised by Jeff Sessions and Stephen Miller as the major component of their Immigration Manifesto. The subsequent "zero tolerance" program of separating children from their parents was designed to instill fear among potential families attempting to immigrate to the United States. It was an effort to stem the previous flood of children fleeing the horrors and violence, extreme poverty, and gangs in Central America. The Sessions/Miller plan was to greatly restrict the availability of legal entry points, causing massive logjams forcing asylum seekers to enter elsewhere which was illegal. In April 2017, AG Jeff Sessions directed federal prosecutors along the southwest border to prioritize the prosecution of immigration-related offenses. Here, a parent or parents caught entering "illegally" would be charged with a misdemeanor for a first offense and a felony if caught again attempting an "improper re-entry." Either offense warranted the immediate arrest and detention, and usual deportation, of the parent while the underage child or children, who were not charged with a crime, would be forcefully removed from their parent(s) without either party knowing where the child would be detained. The "Zero Tolerance" separation program was so successful that it overwhelmed the ORR leading to often squalid living conditions let along the psychological trauma associated with this process.

> THE TRUMP ADMINISTRATION'S FAMILY SEPARATION POLICY: TRAMUA, DESTRUCTION, AND CHAOS.
>
> VI. Conclusion
> While we may never know the full extent of the damage inflicted by the Trump Administration's family separation policy, it is evident—as a result of this investigation and public reporting—that it was driven by an Administration that was willfully blind to its cruelty and determined to go to unthinkable extremes to deliver on political promises and stop migrants fleeing violence from seeking protection in the United States. As illustrated in this report:
>
> - Within weeks of President Trump's inauguration, the Administration began formulating a plan to separate parents from their children as a means to deter migration.
> - Before a formal policy had even been developed, the Administration was accelerating family separations. By March 2017, the number of separated children transferred to ORR custody had increased by nearly 900 percent, as compared to November 2016.
> - In July 2017, without warning, the Administration implemented a family separation pilot program in the El Paso Border Patrol Sector. The pilot program lasted five months and resulted in hundreds of additional children being taken from their parents and placed in ORR custody.
> - During the pilot program, the Administration discovered that it was unable to track separated family members in a way that would facilitate eventual reunification.
> - Knowing this, and without doing anything to address the tracking systems employed by deferral agencies, the Administration chose to expand the policy nationwide in May 2018.
> - To make matters worse, the Administration failed to provide advance notice of the policy to front line agents and officers, which caused unnecessary chaos and inconsistent implementation of the policy across border sectors.
> - When judicial intervention and political pressure eventually resulted in the end of the policy, the lack of interagency cooperation and preparedness was laid bare by the inability of the Administration to quickly reunite separated parents and children.
>
> As a result of this dark chapter in our nation's history, hundreds of migrant children may never be reunited with their parents.[31]

On "Day One" of his prudency, Joe Biden used Executive Orders to reverse three major immigration policies of the Trump era: restrictions on U.S. entry for seven Muslim-majority countries, ceased Trump's expansion of immigration enforcement within the country, and halted construction of the border wall by terminating Trump's National Emergency Declaration used to fund it. Like previous administrations, Executive Orders remain valid only during the President's term in office and can easily be overturned by an incoming president. Legislation is the preferred route to a more humane and ethical immigration policy in America.

The COVID Crises

The unexpected coronavirus shook the world in early 2020 disrupting world economies and political systems including that of the Trump Administration. There is a strong argument that President Donald J. Trump could have won a second four-year term based merely on the strength of the economy. But the U.S. shutdown, like that throughout most of the world, devastated the economy. That, and the President's lax and often contentious and seemingly dismissive approach to the virus, which he labeled the "China Flu," contributed greatly to his eventual defeat. Something that is both deadly and invisible challenges the status quo including individual belief systems leading to a collective malaise manifested by depression and anxiety—conditions that are likely to lead to anomie. How a society addresses a pandemic is crucial to both its control and the collective response of its citizens. Unchecked rumors, especially those promoted by the political leadership, can exacerbate existing social divisions and, by doing so, the effective containment of a pandemic. It is foolhardy to subscribe to the theory that a diabolic power purposefully created and let loose the coronavirus for the purpose of world dominance given that it would infect their society as well.

Mustering support for fighting an unseen enemy is contingent upon the degree of social solidarity at the time of the crises. As previously mentioned in the book, group solidarity is based on shared belief systems that provides answers to the otherwise unanswerable existential questions regarding life and death, essence and being—our existence and purpose. Usually, these belief mythologies can neither be proven nor disproved often relying on shared collective delusions. Ostensibly, when these belief systems are suddenly challenged by an inexplicit crisis, like an invisible virus, chaos results. Political leaders often take advantage of the chaos in order to attempts to further enhance their authority like the military coup in Myanmar in February 2021. Donald J. Trump attempted a similar coup in his efforts to overturn the will of the American people in the 2020 elections. Unwittingly, the Trump insurrection, instead, drew attention to the simmering racial and political strains long latent within American society—those factors supportive of White supremacy and insidious institutional/systemic racism. Here, labeling and symbols help define one's stance in America's 21st-century civil war.

People caught up in chaotic situations, like a seemingly unending pandemic, seek new alliances and assurances to allay their fears and anxieties over the disruption to the status quo. Some will join the "deniers" who see the COVID-19 crisis as a hoax or at least overstated. Others will follow the science and comply with universally accepted health standards like social distancing, constant hand sanitation, and mask wearing, especially in public. Mask wearing has come to symbolize in which camp people belong. Politicizing mask wearing became a rallying call epitomized by President Trump himself as well as by other "populist" leaders. Unfortunately, politicizing the pandemic merely served to prolong its existence allowing for it to mutate into more dangerous and contagious strains posing serious challenges to the massive vaccination effort worldwide. Trump's politicizing of the COVID crisis had an impact on the massive economic rescue packet passed by Congress by virtue of his action to curtail independent oversight measure built into these packets fueling more public distrust and furthering the social divide in America. While many small businesses, notably those run by minorities, were basically shut out of these recovery programs, large corporations, powerful law firms, and well-endowed colleges and universities, including Ivy League schools, received government payments. In February 2021, U.S. Senator Elizabeth Warren of Massachusetts called attention to the payout provided General Healthcare, one of the large nursing home chain in the United States where excessive COVID deaths occurred, providing its CEO with a $5.2 million bonus. The nursing home COVID death rate far exceeded that of other countries. While obviously not deliberate, these facilities were slow to stem the tide of excessive deaths among its residents.[32]

The coronavirus while universally pervasive, its degree of infection, including death, varies according to certain social metrics, including exposure, age, existing health conditions, rural/urban factors, gender, and race and ethnicity. The wide distribution of vaccines is paramount in reaching "herd immunity" across the globe. Nonetheless, privileged entitlement, regardless of social status (nationality, gender, race/ethnicity, religion, political affiliation), is often expressed in terms of inalienable rights and privilege that supersedes others. Nationalism and elitism play a role in the availability of vaccine coverage. To illustrate, Israel offers the vaccine Moderna to any citizen aged 16 or older with the expectation of vaccinating everyone aged 50 or older by mid-February 2021. Yet, some five million Palestinians in adjacent West Bank and Garza communities await the promise of the Russian Sputnik vaccine. Clearly, groups living in close proximity of each other need to have most of their members vaccinated in order to curtail the continued spread of COVID and its mutations. There are numerous examples where the privileged cut to the front of the line. With front-line health-care workers slated for vaccinations, some hospitals and nursing homes have slipped in administrators and even board members into that pool. In Canada, a wealthy couple chartered a plane to the Yukon in an attempt to pass themselves as health-care workers in order to receive vaccines slated for the highly vulnerable Indigenous White River First Nation tribe.

Donald J. Trump's "America First" ethnocentrism put the United States at odds with the World Health Organization (WHO) and its shared vaccine consortium—COVID-19 Vaccine Global Access Facility (COVAX). He was not the first to prioritize health-care preventive measures. This practice extends back to White contact where Black slaves and American Indians suffered most from virulent contagious diseases up until the 20th century. Little is documented on the death of Black and Indian slaves during the colonial era from any of the major European colonizers—Britain, Spain, or France. It is estimated that contagious diseases unwittingly brought to the Americas contributed to the death of millions of Indigenous peoples decimating their tribes and cultures.[33]

The new Biden Administration has reversed many of the Trump era isolationist and nationalistic policies including rejoining the WHO. COVID has run rampant in Indian Country, that vast array of tribes and bands under federal care, a situation that should not have been allowed to happen if Public Health Services (PHS), notably Indian Health Service (IHS), was properly funded and staffed as required by treaty obligations. Some 400,000 deaths are attributed to the COVID-19 epidemic within a year's time of its first U.S. contact, a statistic coinciding with the inauguration of President Biden on January 20, 2021. This is considered to be a gross undercount of the actual COVID-related death. Even then, many survivors continue to suffer devastating side effects, some lifelong. Given this scenario, it is an ethical imperative that the most vulnerable, in America and worldwide, be given vaccine priority.

The degree of trauma related to the pandemic is contingent upon how we experienced its effects. Health-care providers who spent long hours treating victims and witnessing their sufferings and death are strong candidates for post-traumatic stress disorder (PTSD). Those whose loved ones died alone without being able to say "good by" will also be left with an indelible scar on their psyche. How the coronavirus evolved is also a critical factor in how we perceive the crisis.

In February 2020, rumors circulated about a new severe acute respiratory syndrome (SARS)-type virus emerging from China, but there were no major efforts to curtain it by restricting travel per se because it was not yet considered to be a pandemic. On March 1, a number of us serving on international commissions relevant to reconciliation efforts following the Bosnian war, flew to Banja Luka for a two-week session. I flew from Boston, Massachusetts, to Frankfort, Germany, and then to Belgrade, Serbia, where a number of us were transported via car to Bosnia. Other commission members traveled from Japan, Tasmania, Nigeria, Israel, Austria, Germany, Italy, Russia, and Serbia. We met in a secure closed facility without mask or social distancing protocols. Then, suddenly the commissions were terminated, and there was a rush to get us back home on March 13. Our original flights out of Bosnia were no longer available even flights to Serbia or Germany. International flights were also being cancelled especially to the United Kingdom and Canada. On March 14, I was driven to Belgrade with a lengthy border congestion of miles of tractor trailers waiting to pass customs. I was booked on an early flight to Istanbul, Turkey, on March 15 and then embarked on a nine-hour flight back to Boston arriving late afternoon. Serbia closed its borders the next day (March 16) compelling everyone 65 or older to shelter-in-place. The coronavirus was now seen as a pandemic. On arrival at Boston-Logan, we all had our passports confiscated and herded into a large room—again with no masks provided (I was one of the few who had my own mask) and obviously no social distancing. I was included among the thousands of college students forced to return home from their spring semester abroad. Eventually, we were processed and asked questions relevant to our potential exposure and our current health status. Shortly upon arrival home to New Hampshire, I learned of the COVID death of our Italian colleague from the commission conference. His death was followed by the COVID deaths of two long-time American Indian colleagues (one from New Mexico and the other from the Eastern Band of Cherokee Indians). These events prefaced my personal COVID experience coloring my perspective on the pandemic and its impact on those within my social cohorts in particular and society in general.

Notes

1 See *Webster's Ninth New Collegiate Dictionary.* Springfield, MA: Merriam-Webster, Inc., Publishers, p. 689.
2 *Ibid.,* p. 628.
3 DSM-5, 2013. *Desk Reference to the Diagnostic Criteria from DSM-5.* Washington, DC: American Psychiatric Publishing, p. 327.
4 See Myers, D. 2002. Attributing Causality: To the Person or the Situation. *Social Psychology* (7th ed.). Boston, MA: McGraw-Hill, pp. 80–103.
5 *Ibid.,* pp. 300–322.
6 See Alterman, E. 2004. *When Presidents Lie: A History of Official Deception and Its Consequences.* New York, NY: Viking/the Penguin Group.
7 *Ibid.,* p. 1.
8 *Ibid.,* pp. 21, 22.
9 See Congressional Bills 116th Congress; from the U.S. Government Publishing Office: H. Res. 755 Enrolled Bill (ENR).
10 See *The Constitution of the United States of America.* Carlisle, MA: Applewood Books, p. 1.
11 *Ibid.*
12 *Ibid.*
13 See Resendez, A. 2016. *The Other Slavery: The Uncovered Story of Indian Enslavement in America.* Boston, MA: Houghton Mifflin Harcourt, p. 303.
14 *Ibid.,* pp. 295, 314.
15 Op. cit., 10.
16 See Woodward, B. 2018. *Fear: Trump in the White House.* New York, NY: Simon & Schuster.

17 See Silk, M. 2020. William Barr, a Catholic, Went Out of His Way to Use the Death Penalty (and Defy Church Teaching). *America: The Jesuit Review*, Politics & Society News. New York, NY: Published by the Catholic Church (December 23).

18 *Ibid.*, p. 1.

19 *Ibid.*

20 See Crary, D. (AP National Writer). 2021. Some Churchgoers Feel Shut Out by White Leaders. *Concord Monitor Religion*. Concord, NH (January 29), p. B3.

21 See CDC. 2021. Mortality. National Vital Statistics System, National Center for Health Statistics. *Centers for Disease Control and Prevention*. Washington, DC (2019 date set).

22 See *Atkins v. Virginia* 536 U.S. 304 (2002) U.S. Supreme Court; *Roper v. Simmons,* 543 U.S. 551 (2005) U.S. Supreme Court.

23 See USSC 2021. Sotomayor, J. Dissenting. *SUPREME COURT OF THE UNITED STATES. United States v. Dustin John Higgs*: On petition for Writ of Certiorari before judgment to the United States Court of Appeals for the Fourth Circuit and application to vacate stay. 592 U.S. (2021) No. 20-927 20A134).

24 See Woodward, 2018, op. cit. 16; Woodward, B. 2020. *RAGE*. New York, NY: Simon & Schuster.

25 See text of President Donald J. Trump's Address to the Nation on the Crisis of the Border, Washington, DC: January 8, 2019, 9:01 P.M. EST–9:11 P.M. EST.

26 See French, L.A., & Manzanarez, M. 2019. *Borders and Immigration: The Geo*Politics of Marketplace Demands and Ethnic Relations.* Lanham, MD: Lexington Books, Rowman & Littlefield, p. 158.

27 See Cohen, R., & Dees, M. 2018. A Year-End Report: Fighting hate and injustice in Trump era, *SPLC Report*. Vol. 48 (4) (Winter), pp. 1, 8.

28 *Ibid.*, Trump's immigration policy comes straight from hate group's playbook, p. 3.

29 See Mills, K.I. 2020. American Psychological Association Calls for Immediate Halt to Sharing Immigrant Youths' Confidential Psychotherapy Notes with ICE, *APA Press Release.* (February 17): apa.org/news/press/releases/2020/02/sharing-therapy-notes.

30 See Merchant, N. (Associated Press). 2020. Immigration—Judge: Stop Deporting Kids. *Concord Monitor* (November 19), p. B2; Dearing, J., & Burke, G. (Associated Press). 2020. Pence Closed Borders against CDC's Opinion. *Concord Monitor* (October 4), p. A2.

31 See Nadler, J. 2020. *The Trump Administration's Family Separation Policy: Trauma, Destruction, and Chaos.* Majority Staff Report, Committee on the Judiciary U.S. House of Representatives (October). Washington, DC: U.S. Congress.

32 See Englund, W. (*The Washington Post*). 2021. Warren Calls Genesis Healthcare Executive Bonus Act of "Greed." *Concord Monitor* (February 3), p. B2.

33 See French, L.A., & Manzanarez, M. 2017. *North American Border Conflicts: Race, Politics, and Ethics.* Boca Raton, FL: CRC Press/Taylor and Francis Group, pp. 1–5.

SELECTED BIBLIOGRAPHY

Abood, R.R., & Brushwood, D.B. 1994. *Pharmacy Practice and the Law.* Gaithersburg, MD: Aspen Publishers, Inc.

ACLU. 2020. *The Constitution of the United States of America.* Washington, DC: American Civil Liberties Union. www.aclu.org.

Adi, A., & Mathbout, M. 2018. The Duty to Protect: Four Decades after *Tarasoff. American Journal of Psychiatry Residents' Journal,* (April, 2018), pp. 6–8.

Alexander, L. 1949. Medical Science under Dictatorship. *The New England Journal of Medicine,* Vol. 241 (2), pp. 39–47.

Alterman, E. 2004. *When Presidents Lie: A History of Official Deception and Its Consequences.* New York, NY: Viking: The Penguin Group.

Amnesty International. 2006. *Below the Radar: Secret Flights to Torture and "Disappearance."* Amnesty International Report (April 5). London: Amnesty International.

Anderson, J.D. 1988. *The Education of Blacks in the South, 1860–1935.* Chapel Hill, NC: University of North Carolina Press.

Annas, G.J., & Grodin, M.A. (eds.). 1992. *Nazi Doctors and the Nuremberg Code: Human Rights in Human Experimentation.* New York, NY: Oxford University Press.

APA. 2005. *Report of the American Psychological Association Presidential Task Force on Psychological Ethics and National Security (PENS Report).* Washington, DC: American Psychological Association (June).

APA. 2012. A Resolution to Annul the APA's PENS Report. *Coalition for an Ethical Psychology.* www.ethicalpsychology.org.

APA. 2021. *Ethical Principles of Psychologists and Code of Conduct.* Washington, DC: American Psychological Association. www.APA.org.

Barnes, H.E., & Teeters, N.K. 1959. *New Horizons in Criminology* (3rd ed.). Englewood Cliffs, NJ: Prentice-Hall, Inc.

Bear, J., & Bear, M. 2000. *College Degrees by Mail & Internet.* Berkeley, CA: Ten Speed Press.

Becker, H.S. 1963. *Outsiders: Studies in the Sociology of Deviance.* New York, NY: The Free Press.

Begg, M. 2006. *Enemy Combatant: My Imprisonment at Guantanamo, Bagram, Kandaber.* New York, NY: New Press.

Benton-Cohen, K. 2018. *Inventing the Immigration Problem: The Dillingham Commission and Its Legacy.* Cambridge, MA: Harvard University Press.

Berry, J., & Renner, G. 2004. *Vows of Silence: The Abuse of Power in the Papacy of John Paul II.* New York, NY: The Free Press.

Black, E. 2003. *War against the Weak: Eugenics and America's Campaign to Create a Master Race.* New York, NY: Four Walls Eight Windows.

Blum, G.B. 1986. *Bad Karma: A True Story of Obsession and Murder*. New York, NY: Atheneum.

Bond, H.M. 1966. *The Education of the Negro in the American Social Order*. New York, NY: Octagon Books.

Bovard, J. 2003. *Terrorism and Tyranny: Trampling Freedom, Justice, and Peace to Rid the World of Evil*. New York, NY: Palgrave Macmillan.

Boxill, B.R. 1992. *Blacks and Social Justice*. Totowa, NJ: Rowman & Littlefield.

Breyer, C.R., Reeves, D.C., Cushwa, P.K., & Wong, C.D. 2020. *Retroactivity & Recidivism: The Drugs Minus Two Amendment*. Washington, DC: U.S. Sentencing Commission.

Brooks, R.L. (ed.). 1999. *When Sorry Isn't Enough: The Controversy over Apologies and Reparations for Human Injustices*. New York, NY: New York University Press.

Brunner, B. 2009. *The Tuskegee Syphilis Experiment*. Vancouver, BC, Canada: S.O.S. Society of Syphilitics . www.tushegee.edu\global\story.

Buck v. Bell, 274 U.S. 200, 205, No. 292, U.S. Supreme Court, 1927.

Bullock, H.A. 1967. *The History of Negro Education in the South from 1619 to the Present*. Cambridge, MA: Harvard University Press.

Burrough, B. 2004. *Public Enemies: America's Greatest Crime Wave and the Birth of the FBI: 1933–34*. New York, NY: Penguin Books.

Cartwright, S.A. 1851. Report on the Diseases and Physical Peculiarities of the Negro Race. *The New Orleans Medical and Surgical Journal*, (May), pp. 691–715.

CDC. *Syphilis Study at Tuskegee: The Tuskegee Timeline*. Washington, DC: The Center for Disease Control and Prevention; U.S. Public Health Service. www.cdc/gov/tuskegee/timeline.htm.

Charles, A., & Draper, H. 2012. "Equivalence of Care" in Prison Medicine: Is Equivalence of Process the Right Measure of Equity? *Journal of Medical Ethics*, Vol. 38 (4), pp. 215–218.

Clark, K.B. 1967. *Dark Ghetto: Dilemma of Social Power*. Middletown, CT: Wesleyan University Press.

Cohn, M. 2007. *Cowboy Republic: Six Ways the Bush Gang Has Defied the Law*. Sausalito, CA: PoliPoint Press.

Cook, J.L. 1973. *The Advisor: The Phoenix Program in Vietnam*. Philadelphia, PA: Dorrance & Company.

Cosby, W.H., Jr. 1976. *An Integration of the Visual Media via "Fat Albert and the Cosby Kids" into the Elementary School Curriculum as a Teaching Aid and Vehicle to Achieve Increased Learning* (Doctoral Dissertation). Amherst, MA: University of Massachusetts (#AAT7706369).

Coser, L.A. 1955. *The Function of Social Conflict*. Glencoe, IL: The Free Press.

Coser, L.A. 1956. *Continuities in the Study of Social Conflict*. Glencoe, IL: The Free Press.

Coser, L.A. 1977. *Masters of Sociological Thought: Ideas in Historical and Social Context*. New York, NY: Harcourt, Brace and Jovanovich.

Cremin, L. 1961. *The Transformation of the School*. New York, NY: Vintage.

Cullather, N. 1999. *Secret History: The CIA's Classified Account of Its Operations in Guatemala, 1952–1954*. Palo Alto, CA: Stanford University Press.

Daniel, C. 1987. *Chronicle of the 29th Century*. New York, NY: Chronicle Publications, Inc.

Dewey, J. 1961. *Democracy and Education*. New York, NY: Macmillan.

Dollard, J. 1937. *Caste and Class in a Southern Town*. New Haven, CT: Yale University Press.

Donald, D.H., Baker, J.H., & Holt, M.F. 2001. *The Civil War and Reconstruction*. New York, NY: W.W. Norton & Company.

Draper, R. 2007. *Dead Certain: The Presidency of George W. Bush*. New York, NY: Free Press.

Drug Amendments Act of 1962. 2008. *Enrolled Acts and Resolutions of Congress, Compiled 1789–2008*. Washington, DC: U.S. National Archives and Records Administration.

Durkheim, E. 1949. *The Division of Labor in Society* (Simpson, G. trans.). Glencoe, IL: The Free Press.

Durkheim, E. 1950. *The Rules of Sociological Methods* (Solovay, S., & Mueller, J., trans.). Glencoe, IL: The Free Press.

Durkheim, E. 1951. *Suicide* (Spaulding, J.A., & Simpson, G., trans.). Glencoe, IL: The Free Press.

Edgerton, J.E., & Campbell, R.J. (eds.). 1994. *American Psychiatry Glossary* (7th ed.). Washington, DC: American Psychiatric Press, Inc.

Erikson, K.T. 1966. *Wayward Puritans: A Study in the Sociology of Deviance*. New York, NY: John Wiley & Sons.

Erikson, K.T. 1976. *Everything in Its Path*. New York, NY: Simon and Schuster.

Erikson, K.T. 1994. *A New Species of Trouble: The Human Experience of Modern Disasters*. New York, NY: W.W. Norton.

Evans, S. 2008. *U.S. Marines and Irregular Warfare, 1898–2007: Anthology and Selected Bibliography*. Quantico, VA: Marine Corps University Press.

Folly, M. 2014. Phoenix Program, *Historical Dictionary of U.S. Diplomacy during the Cold War*. Lanham, MD: Rowman & Littlefield Publishers.

French, L.A. 1987. *Psychocultural Change and the American Indian: An Ethnohistorical Analysis*. New York, NY: Garland.

French, L.A. 1994. *The Winds of Injustice: American Indians and the U.S. Government*. New York, NY: Garland.

French, L.A. 1995. Treating the Dangerous Sexual Offender. *Sexual Issues in Counseling & Therapy* (Lesson #6). Long Island, NY: The Hatherleigh Company.

French, L.A. 2003. *Native American Justice*. Chicago, IL: Burnham, Inc.; Lexington Books.

French, L.A. 2007. *Legislating Indian Country: Significant Milestones in Transforming Tribalism*. New York, NY: Peter Lang.

French, L.A. 2010. *Running the Border Gauntlet: The Mexican Migrant Controversy*. Santa Barbara, CA: Praeger, ABC-CLIO, LLC.

French, L.A. 2014. *Frog Town: Portrait of a French Canadian Parish in New England*. Lanham, MD: University Press of America.

French, L.A. 2018. *The History of Policing America: From Militias and Military to the Law Enforcement of Today*. Lanham, MD: Rowman & Littlefield.

French, L.A., & Nikolic-Novakovic, L. 2012. *War Trauma and Its Aftermath: An International Perspective on the Balkan and Gulf Wars*. Lanham, MD: University Press of America.

French, L.A., & Manzanarez, M. 2017. *North American Border Conflicts: Race, Politics, and Ethics*. Boca Raton, FL: CRC/Taylor & Francis Group.

French, L.A., & Manzanarez, M. 2019. *Borders and Immigration: The Geo-Politics of Marketplace Demands and Ethnic Relations*. Lanham, MD: Lexington Books.

Freud, S. 1927; 1964. *The Future of an Illusion* (Robson-Scott, W.D., trans.; Strachely, J., ed.). Garden City, NY: Doubleday Anchor.

Galton, F. 1869. *Hereditary Genius: An Inquiry into Its Laws and Consequences*. London, England: Macmillan.

Garcia, J.R. 1980. *Operation Wetback: The Mass Deportation of Mexican Undocumented Workers in 1954*. Westport, CT: Greenwook Press.

Garfield, H. 1949. Research Note in Inter- and Intra-Racial Homicides. *Social Forces*, Vol. 27, pp. 381–396.

Gentry, G. 1991. *J. Edgar Hoover: The Man and the Secrets*. New York, NY: W.W. Norton & Company.

Ginsburg, R. 1962. *100 Years of Lynchings*. New York, NY: Lancer Books.

Goldhagen, D.J. 1996. *Hilter's Willing Executioners: Ordinary Germans and the Holocaust*. New York, NY: Alfred A. Knopf.

Goldman, C.A., & Massey, W.F. 2001. *The PhD Factory*. Bolton, MA: Anker Publishing Company.

Goldsmith, J.L. 2007. *The Terror Presidency: Law and Judgment Inside the Bush Administration*. New York, NY: Norton.Gonzalez, J. 2000. *Harvest of Empire: A History of Latinos in America*. New York, NY: Viking.

Good, H., & Teller, J. 1967. *History of American Education*. New York, NY: Macmillan.

Goode, E. 1969. Marijuana and the Politics of Reality. *Journal of Health and Social Behavior*, Vol. 10, pp. 83–94.

Grant, A. 1995. *No End to Grief: Indian Residential Schools in Canada*. Winninpeg, Manitoba, Canada: Pemmican.

Green, D.H. 1948. Ethics Governing the Services of Prisoners as Subjects in Medical Experiments: Report of the Committee Appointed by Governor Dwight H. Green of Illinois. *Journal of the American Medical Association (JAMA)*, Vol. 136, pp. 457–458.

Greenberg, K.J., & Dratel, J.L. (eds.). 2005. *The Torture Papers: The Road to Abu Ghraib*. Cambridge, England: Cambridge University Press.

Greene, J.M. 2003. *Justice at Dachau*. New York, NY: Broadway Books.

Greenfield, R. 2006. *Timothy Leary: A Biography*. Boston, MA: Houghton-Mifflin Harcourt.

Grey, S. 2006. *Ghost Plane: The True Story of the CIA Torture Program*. New York, NY: St. Martin's Press.

Guenter, L. 1978. *America in Vietnam*. New York, NY: Oxford University Press.

Guimaraes, A.S. 1999. *The Catholic Church and Homosexuality*. Charlotte, NC: Tan Books and Publications.

Gwynne, S.C. 2010. *Empire of the Summer Moon: Quanah Parker and the Rise and Fall of the Comanches—The Most Powerful Indian Tribe in American History*. New York, NY: Scribne.

Hatfield, J.H. 2002. *Fortunate Son: George W. Bush and the Making of an American President*. New York, NY: Soft Skull Press.

Havinghurst, R. 1968. *Comparative Perspectives on Education*. Boston, MA: Little, Brown.

Hayes, S. 2019. Sackler Family Philanthropy: Museums Cut Long Standing Ties. *Time* (April 8), p. 11.

Heckscher, A. 1996. *A Brief History of St. Paul's School, 1856–1996*. Concord, NH: St. Paul School Publication.

Immerman, R.H. 1982. *The CIA in Guatemala: The Foreign Policy of Intervention*. Austin, TX: University of Texas Press.

International Military Tribunal. 1945–1946. *In the Matter of the United States of America, the French Republic, the United Kingdom of Great Britain and Northern Ireland, and the Union of Soviet Socialist Republics versus Hermann Wilhelm Goering, et al.* Washington, DC: United States Government Printing Office.

Jackson, H. 1917. *A Century of Dishonor: A Sketch of the United States Government's Dealings with Some of the Indian Tribes*. Boston, MA: Little, Brown, & Company.

Jenkins, P. 2001. *Pedophiles and Priests: Anatomy of a Contemporary Crisis*. New York, NY: Oxford University Press.

Jennings, F. 1990. *Empire of Fortune: Crowns, Colonies, and Tribes in the Seven Years War in America*. New York, NY: W.W. Norton.

Johnson, B.H. 2003. *Revolution in Texas: How a Forgotten Rebellion and Its Bloody Suppression Turned Mexicans into Americans*. New Haven, CT: Yale University Press.

Jones, I. 2010. *The Human Factor: Inside the CIA's Dysfunctional Intelligence Culture*. New York, NY: Encounter Books.

Jones, J. 1981. *Bad Blood: The Tuskegee Syphilis Experiment*. New York, NY: The Free Press.Katz, J. 1972. *Experimentation with Human Beings*. New York, NY: Russell Sage Foundation.

Kefauver Harris Amendment. 1962. *Federal Food, Drug, and Cosmetic Act—Drug Efficacy Amendment*. 21 U.S.C. Food and Drugs; Public Law 87–781; 76 Stat. 788–789, October 10, 1962.

Khan, S.R. 2011. *Privilege: The Making of an Adolescent Elite at St. Paul's School*. Princeton, NJ: Princeton University Press.

Kinzer, S., & Schlesinger, S. 1999. *Bitter Fruit: The Story of the American Coup in Guatemala*. Cambridge, MA: Harvard University Press.

Kliebard, H.M. 1969. *Religion and Education in America: A Documentary History*. Scranton, PA: International Textbook Company.

Kondro, W. 1998. Canada Apologies to Native People Who Suffered Abuse. *The Lancet*, Vol. 351 (9097), p. 194.

Lesley, G. 2004. *The School of the Americas: Military Training and Political Violence in the Americas*. Durham. NC: Duke University Press.

Linton, R.J. 1986. *The Nazi Doctors*. New York, NY: Basic Books.

Lipstadt, D.E. 1993. *Denying the Holocaust: The Growing Assault on Truth and Memory*. New York, NY: The Free Press.

Mackey, C., & Miller, G. 2004. *The Interrogators: Inside the Secret War Against Al Queda*. New York, NY: Little, Brown.

Margulies, J. 2006. *Guantanamo and the Abuse of Presidential Power*. New York, NY: Simon & Schuster.

Marks, H. 1997. *The Progress of Experiment: Science and Therapeutic Reform in the United States, 1900–1990*. New York, NY: Russell Sage Foundation.

Martinez, O. 2016. *A History of Violence: Living and Dying in Central America* (Washington, J.B., & Ugaz, D., trans.). London, England: Verso.

May, R.E. 2002. *Manifest Destiny's Underworld: Filibustering in Antebellum America*. Chapel Hill, NC: University of North Carolina Press.

Mayer, J. 2008. *The Dark Side: The Inside Story of How the War on Terror Turned into a War on American Ideals*. New York, NY: Doubleday.McCoy, A. 2006. *A Question of Torture: CIA Interrogation from the Cold War to the War on Terror*. New York, NY: Metropolitan Books.

McKelvey, T. 2007. *Monstering: Inside America's Policy of Secret Interrogations and Torture in the Terror War*. New York, NY: Carroll & Graf.

Meijer, M. (ed.). 2001. *Dealing with Human Rights: Asian and Western Views on the Value of Human Rights*. Oxford, England: World View Publishing.

Melton, G.B., Petrila, J., Plytghress, N.C., & Slobogin, C. 1997. The Duty to Protect the Public (Tarasoff). *Psychological Evaluations for the Courts: A Handbook for Mental Health Professionals and Lawyers* (2nd ed.). New York, NY: The Guilford Press, pp. 76–77.

Meriam, L. 1928. *The Problem of Indian Administration*. Baltimore, MD: Johns Hopkins Press.
Merton, R.K. 1968. *Social Theory and Social Structure*. New York, NY: The Free Press.
Milgram, S. 1974. *Obedience to Authority*. New York, NY: Harper and Row.
Miller, N.E. 1941. The frustration-aggression hypothesis. *Psychological Review*, Vol. 48, pp. 337–342.
Mitchell, J., & B. Harlow. 2016. *Enhanced Interrogation*. New York, NY: Penguin Random House.
Mitford, J. 1973. *Kind & Unusual Punishment: The Prison Business*. New York, NY: Alfred A. Knopf.
Morsink, J. 1999. *The Universal Declaration of Human Rights*. Philadelphia, PA: University of Pennsylvania Press.
Murdal, G. 1944. *The American Dilemma: The Negro Problem in American Democracy*. New York, NY: Harper.
Nash, G. 1974. *Red, White and Black: The Peoples of Early America*. Englewood Cliffs, NJ: Prentice-Hall.
Novak, D.A. 1978. *The Wheel of Servitude: Black Forced Labor after Slavery*. Lexington, KY: University Press of Kentucky.
Otterman, M. 2007. *American Torture: From the Cold War to Abu Ghraib and Beyond*. Melbourne, Australia: Melbourne University Press.
Overby, A. 1972. Discrimination in the Administration of Justice. *Race, Crime and Justice* (Reasons, C.E., ed.). Pacific Palisades, CA: Goodyear Publishing Company, pp. 264–276.
Palmer, S.H. 1998. *The Universities Today: Scholarship, Self-Interest, and Politics*. Lanham, MD: University Press of America.
Pareto, V. 1935. *The Mind and Society* (Livingston, A., trans.). New York, NY: Harcourt, Brace & Company.
Park, R.E. 1964. *Race and Culture*. New York, NY: The Free Press.Peltzman, S. 1973. An Evaluation of Consumer Protection Legislation: The 1962 Drug Amendments. *The Journal of Political Economy*, Vol. 81 (5), p. 1051.
Peters, E. 1966. *Torture*. Philadelphia, PA: Pennsylvania Press.
Peterson, V.S., & Runya, A.S. 1993. *Global Gender Issues*. Boulder, CO: Westview Press.
Petrunik, M., & Deutschmann, L. 2007. The Exclusion-Inclusion Spectrum in State and Community Responses to Sex Offenders in Anglo-American and European Jurisdictions. *International Journal of Offender Therapy and Comparative Criminology*, Vol. 20 (10), pp. 1–21.
Phayer, M. 1965. *The Catholic Church and the Holocaust, 1930–1965*. Bloomington, IN: Indiana University Press.
Piaget, J. 1970. *Psychology and Epistemology*. New York, NY: Viking.
Pratt, R. 1964. *Battlefield and Classroom* (Utley, R., ed.). New Haven, CT: Yale University Press.
Prucha, F. 1990. *Documents of United States Indian Policy*. Lincoln, NE: University of Nebraska Press.
Quinney, R. 1974. *Critique of Legal Order: Crime Control in Capitalist Society*. Boston, MA: Little, Brown and Company.
Reiter, K. 2009. Experimentation on Prisoners: Persistent Dilemmas in Rights and Regulations. *California Law Review*, Vol. 97, pp. 501–566.
Resendez, A. 2016. *The Other Slavery: The Uncovered Story of Indian Enslavement in America*. Boston, MA: Houghton Mifflin Harcourt.
Reverby, S.M. (ed.). 2000. *Tuskegee's Truths: Rethinking the Tuskegee Syphilis Study*. Chapel Hill, NC: University of North Carolina Press.
Richard, W. 1967. *The Handbook of Prescription Drugs*. New York, NY: Pantheon Books-Random House.
Risen, J. 2006. *State of War: The Secret History of the CIA and the Bush Administration*. New York, NY: Free Press.
Risen, J. 2014. *Pay any Price: Greed, Power, and Endless War*. New York, NY: Houghton, Mifflin Harcourt.Rivers, P.C. 1994. *Alcohol and Human Behavior: Theory, Research, and Practice*. Englewood Cliffs, NJ: Prentice-Hall.
Rodriquez, M.A., & Garcia, R. 2013. First, Do No Harm: The US Sexually Transmitted Disease Experiments in Guatemala. *American Journal of Public Health*, Vol. 103 (12), pp. 2122–2126.
Rorabaugh, W.J. 1979. *The Alcohol Republic: An American Tradition*. New York, NY: Oxford University Press.
Rose, D. 2004. *Guantanamo: The War on Human Rights*. New York, NY: New Press.
Rousseau, J.J. 1767. *A Thesis on the Social Compact*. London, England: T. Becket & P.A. DeHondt.
Scheibeck, H., et al. 1976. *Report on Indian Education, Task Force Five*. Washington, DC: U.S. Government Printing Office.
Schirmer, J. 2000. *The Guatemalan Military Project: A Violence called Democracy*. Philadelphia, PA: University of Pennsylvania Press.
Schmidt, U. 2004. *Justice at Nuremberg: Leo Alexander and the Nazi Doctors' Trial*. New York, NY: Palgrave Macmillan.

Sehat, D. 2015. *The Jefferson Rule: How the Founding Fathers Became Infallible and Our Politics of Inflexible.* New York, NY: Simon & Schuster.

Seligman, M.E.P. 1975. *Learned Helplessness: On Depression, Development, and Death.* San Francisco, CA: W.H. Freeman.

Seligman, M.E.P. 2018. The Hoffman Report, the Central Intelligence Agency, and the defense of the Nation: A personal view. *Health Psychology Open*, Vol. 5 (2) (July–December). www.ncbi.nlm.nih.gov.

Selye, H. 1976. *The Stress of Life.* New York, NY: McGraw-Hill.

Sheehan, B. 1974. *Seeds of Extinction.* New York, NY: W.W. Norton.

Simmel, G. 1955. *Conflict* (Wolff, K.A., trans.). New York, NY: The Free Press.

Sloan, L. 1979. *History of Marijuana in America.* Indianapolis, IN: Bobbs-Merril.

Sluka, J.A. 1999. *Death Squad: The Anthropology of State Terror.* Philadelphia, PA: University of Pennsylvania Press.

Sorokin, P.A. 1959. *Social and Cultural Mobility.* Glencoe, IL: The Free Press.

Spencer, H. 1874. *The Principles of Sociology.* London, England: Appleton.

Spitz, V. 2005. *Doctors from Hell: The Horrific Account of Nazi Experiments on Humans.* Boulder, CO: Sentient Publications.

Stanaard, D.E. 1992. *American Holocaust: The Conquest of the New World.* New York, NY: Oxford University Press.

Steiner, J., & Brown, R.M. 1927. *The North Carolina Chain Gang.* Chapel Hill, NC: University of North Carolina Press.

Stephanson, A. 1995. *Manifest Destiny.* New York, NY: Hill and Wang.

Stonequist, E. 1937. *The Marginal Man.* New York, NY: Russell and Russell.

Subramanian, S. 2017. Worse Than Tuskegee. *Slate.* eagleeye.umw.edu\2017\02\28\subramanian-published-slate.

Szasz, M.C. 1977. *Education and the American Indian: The Road to Self-Determination since 1928.* Albuquerque, NM: University of New Mexico Press.

Tanielian, Jaycox, L.H. (ed.). 2008. *Invisible Wounds of War: Summary and Recommendations for Addressing Psychological and Cognitive Injuries* (Document No. MG-720/1-CCF). Santa Monica, CA: Rand Corporation.

Taylor, T. 1992. *Anatomy of the Nuremberg Trials.* New York, NY: Alfred A. Knopf.

Terman, L.M. 1916. *The Measurement of Intelligence.* Boston, MA: Houghton Mifflin.

The National Commission on Terrorist Attacks Upon the United. 2004. *The 9/11 Commission Report.* New York, NY: W.W. Norton.

Thorndike, E. 1913. *The Psychology of Learning.* New York, NY: Teachers College Press.

Thorndike, R.M., & Lohman, D.F. 1990. *A Century of Ability Testing.* Chicago, IL: The Riverside Publishing Company.

Tirman, J. 2011. *The Death of Others: The Fate of Civilians in America's Wars.* New York, NY: Oxford University Press.

Tonnies, F. 1957. *Communities and Society* (Loomis, C.P., trans.). East Lansing, MI: Michigan State University Press.

Tsesis, A. (ed.). 2010. *The Promise of Liberty: The History and Contemporary Relevance of the Thirteenth Amendment.* New York, NY: Columbia University Press.

Tyler, T.R., Boeckmann, R.J., Smith, H.J., & Huo, Y.J. 1997. *Social Justice in a Diverse Society.* Boulder, CO: Westview Press.

UN. *Convention against Torture and Other Cruel, Inhuman or Degrading Treatment or Punishment* (Torture Convention). New York, NY: United Nations Treaty Series, Vol. 1465, p. 85. www.reefworld.org/docoid/.

USA. 2009. *Sex-Offenders Registration and Notification Act (SORNA).* www.justice.gov/oig/report/plus/e0901/Final.pdf.

U.S. Congress. 2000. *United States Code Annotated, Title 25, Indians.* St. Paul, MN: West Publishing Company.

Valentine, D. 2014. *The Phoenix Program: America's use of Terror in Vietnam.* New York, NY: Forbidden Bookshelf.

Veblen, T. 1899. *The Theory of the Leisure Class.* New York, NY: Macmillan.

Watson, J.B. 1930. *Behaviorism.* New York, NY: W.W. Norton.

Weber, M. 1930. *The Protestant Ethic and the spirit of Capitalism* (Parsons, T., trans.). London, England: Allen & Unwin.

Weiner, T. 2007. *Legacy of Ashes: The History of the CIA.* New York, NY: Doubleday.

Welsome, E. 1999. *The Plutonium Files: America's Secret Medical Experiments in the Cold War.* New York, NY: Delacorte Press; Penguin-Random House.

Wiegand, T.J. 2007. Captive subjects: Pharmaceutical Testing and Prisoners. *Journal of Medical Toxicology*, Vol. 3 (1) (April), pp. 37–39.

Williams, J.C. 1990. *The Protectors: Anslinger and the Federal Bureau of Narcotics—1930–1962.* Newark, DE: University of Delaware Press.

Woodson, C. 1915. *The Education of the Negro Prior to 1861.* New York, NY: Putnam's.

Woodward, B. 2018. *Fear: Trump in the White House.* New York, NY: Simon & Schuster.

Woodward, B. 2020. *RAGE.* New York, NY: Simon & Schuster.

Young, I.M. 1990. *Justice and the Politics of Differences.* Princeton, NJ: Princeton University Press.

Zimbardo, P. 2007. *The Lucifer Effect: Understanding How Good People Turn Evil.* New York, NY: Random House.

INDEX

For Product Safety Concerns and Information please contact our EU
representative GPSR@taylorandfrancis.com
Taylor & Francis Verlag GmbH, Kaufingerstraße 24, 80331 München, Germany

www.ingramcontent.com/pod-product-compliance
Ingram Content Group UK Ltd.
Pitfield, Milton Keynes, MK11 3LW, UK
UKHW050235200926
475702UK00020B/3038

* 9 7 8 1 0 3 2 1 2 3 3 3 2 *